PE EAVEN

Adventures in Zero Balancing

Exploring Altered States of Consciousness Through Touch

To Jane
best wishes
Gethyn.

Gethyn Williams

Foreword by Fritz Frederick Smith MD

Email: penetratingheaven@gmail.com
www.gethynwilliams.com

Email: theeyeofgabriele@gmail.com

Notice
The information given in this book is intended as a guide for trained practitioners of Zero Balancing. The author does not assume any responsibility for any loss or injury and/or damage to persons or property arising out of, or related to, any use of the material contained in this book. It is the responsibility of the practitioner to use good judgement and determine the best application for their client.

ISBN: 978-1-3999-1306-5

Contents

Part One

Part Two

Foreword

Penetrating Heaven is a charming and educational account by Gethyn Williams of his journey exploring the world of touch and altered states of consciousness. The book describes Williams' investigations searching to understand a formative experience of consciousness he had following a Zero Balancing session. He says: "I have followed my own path [of exploration] – not always clear but ultimately the most rewarding and the best thing I have ever done... I wanted to explore where few others had, and the dark muddy path led me to freedom." Using Zero Balancing as the scaffolding of his search, he highlights ZB principles, his knowledge of Chinese Medicine, Acupuncture, other systems of health and touch, and client feedback to explore a shamanic dimension of Zero Balancing. Based on his belief that the answers to one's problems lie within the self, Williams frames and uses expanded consciousness to help a person search for these answers.

The point, *Penetrating Heaven* (Tian Chong, Gall Bladder 9), is a Window of Heaven or Window of the Sky acupuncture point located on the skull and the one he uses to induce expanded consciousness experiences for the client. "(Penetrating Heaven) opens the client ... to more clarity ... and then answers appear." Williams explains at length how he developed his ideas for using this point, his resultant techniques and the outcomes of the client's experience. His journey is unique, highly educational, well written and well documented. It contains stories of experimentation, successes, failures, logic and intuition, laced with humor and insights.

Penetrating Heaven is an excellent resource for anyone interested in Zero Balancing, expanding their understanding of touch and the use of altered states of consciousness, or for someone before starting off on his or her own personal journey of discovery. Williams' book will find a meaningful place in the library of journeys that explore worlds of health and healing.

Fritz Frederick Smith, MD
Founder of *Zero Balancing*

Preface

In the summer of 2013, after receiving some Zero Balancing from teacher and practitioner Richard Walters, I had a profound inner experience which was to change the direction of my work as a Zero Balancer and Acupuncturist. It inspired me to explore the possibility of using Zero Balancing as a 'springboard' for accessing altered states of consciousness and then to take this further by exploring the effects of conscious touch on Acupuncture points.

My investigations led me to develop a technique for touching Acupuncture points in a certain way, within a Zero Balancing session, which can deeply relax the body and mind and therefore open a person up to access a part of their consciousness that they would not usually experience - a part of them that holds the answers to their innermost questions.

Here I will focus on one particular Acupuncture point: Tian Chong, GB-9, or "Penetrating Heaven".

This book began simply as a session log and clinic journal for me to record my thoughts, ideas and observations, and later included verbal and written feedback from my clients. Later, as I refined my technique, it became an instruction manual to myself as I pieced together clues from each session in order to get a clearer understanding of the altered state experiences and how to work with them.

Part One covers the process of development of my technique of Penetrating Heaven, while Part Two explores how to apply the technique for the purpose of self-development and healing, with examples of client feedback and accounts of their inner journey experiences.

Penetrating Heaven has worked since the first time I tried it but there was a long, gradual process involved in developing and refining my technique, which was challenging at times but ultimately gentle on me and there was always something that propelled me forward. Whenever this path seemed impossible, I was buoyed by client feedback that urged me to keep going.

My clients' journeys have been a part of my own journey of learning to work with and trust my intuition. I have given sessions to people from all walks of life: psychotherapists, artists, musicians, psychologists, hairdressers, writers, teachers, actors and gardeners, all helping me to gather a wide range of perspectives and accounts which I present here to illustrate how these altered state experiences can be useful and transformative.

It is my hope that this book will show that Zero Balancing is more than just bodywork - it is "bodywork for the mind". I would like to encourage other practitioners to try my technique of Penetrating Heaven, which I have woven into the Zero Balancing Protocol, and to test my ideas. I hope to encourage more people to have a session of Zero Balancing and also to train in it. And I hope this book will empower people to realize the potential that is in each one of us to find the answers to life's questions within ourselves, and to inspire more people to explore and pioneer their own path.

Finally, I hope this book will serve as a record of my work so far and tell my story because I believe it is a story that deserves to be told. As one of my regular clients said to me:

"I hope you know how important this work is, Gethyn."

Acknowledgements

Thanks to Dr Fritz Smith, founder of Zero Balancing, for your encouragement, generosity and teaching.

Thanks to Judith Sullivan and Mary Murphy for the Secrets of the Skull workshop.

Thanks to Richard Walters for launching me on my journey.

Thanks to Mike for your willingness to be my first 'test pilot', your patience while I tried out different ideas and experimented on you, and your clear feedback, insights and guidance.

Thanks to Claire for your words of encouragement. You knew the value of this work before I did, and your firm belief in how powerful it can be kept me going through periods of doubt.

Thanks to Gabriele for all our rich conversations over a cuppa at Talk of Tea in Brighton, your comments and suggestions, and later for your proof-reading, high standards of quality, cover design and photography. Thank you for being part of my path.

Thanks to all my clients for your feedback, suggestions and ideas - and for your questions which required me to be clearer in my explanations about how Penetrating Heaven works, all of which helped me to shape this book.

Part One

Introducing Zero Balancing

Zero Balancing (ZB) was created and developed by Dr Fritz Smith, an Osteopath and Acupuncturist. It is a hands-on body/mind system of therapy designed to enhance health by balancing the body's energy and its anatomical structure simultaneously.

Fritz Smith conceptualises two bodies: the energy body and the structural body. Modern science tells us that at a sub-atomic level we are made up of both particles and waves - structure and energy - and Zero Balancing addresses both of these aspects together.

Zero Balancing focuses primarily on the skeleton and the characteristic properties of bone. Thanks to our skeleton we are upright structures, and there is a flow of gravitational energy through us - through our bones - from the crown, spine, sacrum and down to the feet. The resistance to gravity that our bones provide produces a counterflow upward, and it is through bone that this vertical flow is at its most focused and organised.

Fritz saw that this vertical flow of energy down through our skeleton, if likened to a river, would naturally produce eddies or whirlpools at the points of major curvature of the spine, and these also correspond to the chakras - this is where energy meets structure.

In our skeleton, the foundation joints and semi-foundation joints are important because they carry these vertical forces - they are shock absorbers rather than prime movers - and so they hold imbalances, causing us to compensate. We have less conscious awareness and control over these parts of our skeleton. This is where Zero Balancing comes in.

The Zero Balancing Protocol is an inspired sequence which gives the client a guided tour of their own skeleton, addressing the foundation joints and semi-foundation joints including the bones in the lower back and ribs, pelvis, hips, feet, neck, upper back and shoulders, using gentle finger pressure and stretches as an invitation or opportunity to change.

It is now more widely accepted that "our issues are in our tissues" and that emotional trauma can be held in the body, but bones in particular have interesting properties in this regard.

The crystalline structures in bone are piezo-electric, meaning that when bone is subjected to pressure, small electric fields are stimulated throughout the body. Fritz found that bone transmits vibration, and it can store information (as vibration) so that emotions, past trauma and conditioning from early childhood can be stored in our bones as deeply held memory.

Zero Balancing works by introducing a clearer, stronger vibratory field through the bones so that the information (vibration) that is stored there can now be released. The client then becomes less fixed in their old pattern and so they become free to choose and to change. Our body can store tension and trauma, and yet our body can release these by being held. Zero Balancing helps you to feel held in a safe and respectful way.

I found it intriguing that Zero Balancing touches the most physically dense part of us - our bones - yet it can have such a profound effect on the least physical part of us - our mind.

The mind and the body are one, and so it makes sense to work with both simultaneously. Zero Balancing embraces this, which is why I like to think of it as "bodywork for the mind".

I will now give a brief description of some of the basic terms and principles used in Zero Balancing:

DONKEY - The Donkey is the symbolic animal of ZB. If a donkey trusts you then it will lean into you, give itself to you, and if the client trusts me, or rather if their bones trust my hands, they will feel safe and happily give themselves up to my ZB work, and 'lean into' my touch. Donkey is therefore a metaphor for the sub-conscious part of each person that seeks connection. A good "Donkey Connection" between two people promotes trust on an instinctual level.

FRAME - We begin by setting a verbal "Frame" for the session, discussing with the client "What would you like to get out of this session?", without any promise of a specific 'result'. The Frame helps to build rapport and trust and so establishes a good Donkey Connection. A clear Frame provides a structure or energetic 'container' to help focus the session, so what happens in the session will often relate to the Frame or resonate with it in some way.

EVALUATIONS - An integral part of the ZB Protocol is the evaluation of the part of the skeleton on which we are working, by palpating or moving it to determine its quality. Evaluations give the practitioner information and help to 'future pace' the client's Donkey so that the client has a better idea of what to expect and is then more ready and able to let go.

As an Acupuncturist I explored Japanese style Acupuncture, which involves palpation, and I came across the saying: "Diagnosis is treatment and treatment is diagnosis" which suggests that while we palpate or evaluate (mindfully), we are also inviting change. Indeed, I have noticed physical improvements from doing the ZB evaluations on their own.

TOUCH - Zero Balancing involves a certain quality of touch. It is touch with attention, with our awareness in our hands, working with our feeling mind and not our thinking mind.

When we touch a client, we touch both energy and structure together, with an awareness of both simultaneously. Using a sailboat as an analogy, it is where the wind (energy) meets the sail (structure). We aim for just the right amount of tension in the sail to catch the wind.

INTERFACE - We touch at 'Interface', fully engaged but with clear boundaries. At Interface I know where my body ends and where your body begins. And you know where your body ends and my body begins. This feels clear, safe and makes for a good Donkey Connection.

As Fritz says: "Unless I am touched, I don't know who I am". And by knowing who we are, what we are - and what we are not - we are better able to let go of whatever blocks us, and make sense of things as our body reorganises and integrates change.

TOUCH AT INTERFACE means that I put my attention and awareness in my fingers and make a clear bone-to-bone connection with the client. That is to say, I make a connection between the bone in my finger(s) to the client's bone that I am focusing on. That's where my attention is, so I meet the client there.

BLUE LINE - Think of a loose rope connecting two people. When it is pulled tighter, the looseness is taken out and the rope reaches a certain point of tension, allowing communication - we can feel there is something on the other end of the rope. This point is known as the "Blue Line" - where we begin to feel meaningfully engaged with the energy and structure of the other person.

PAUSE - The pause is an inherent part of the rhythm of life. We can pause before taking action, in order to gather, prepare and focus. And we can pause after completing an action (or in between actions), to allow our action to take effect. A pause allows things to happen.

FULCRUM - The Fulcrum is the means by which we do the main 'work' of Zero Balancing. (In physics, a 'fulcrum' is a still point on which a lever can balance to enable movement.) Having previously taken out the looseness to reach the Blue Line and engage properly, we now go further and create a specific field of tension using finger pressure, rotation or stretching in a particular direction.

VECTOR - In describing Fulcrums, a Vector is a force with both magnitude and direction.

HALF MOON VECTOR (HMV) is a special type of Fulcrum with a curved pull, so called because the curved vector is like a crescent half moon. It is typically applied at the feet and neck.

The Fulcrum is held stable to introduce a clearer, stronger field to this part of the body. Holding this constancy, like holding a note in music, for about 3-5 seconds creates a Stillness Point around which the energy of the bone can re-organize itself. Then we insert a Pause.

Clearer, stronger vibratory fields override weaker, less coherent fields, so if the body's energy field is unclear, then it has the opportunity to align to this new clearer, stronger field, creating order where there was disorder. The Fulcrum is an offering, not a manipulation. We simply make an offering and see if the body chooses to accept it and make use of it. Each fulcrum is an invitation or opportunity to change, and so the client has a choice.

Fulcrums should feel good, or sometimes they are 'Hedonic' and "hurt good" - a tension is created between relaxing into yielding to the pleasure and pulling away from the pain. (But adding too much tension or pressure will override any meaningful communication!)

A Fulcrum can be 'local' or 'global'. That is to say, it can affect the bone at the local site where we are working, or it can have a global effect on the whole body or whole person.

Similarly, a Fulcrum can act on the physical aspect (by touch) but also on the mental and emotional aspects of the person, or, as I was to discover, on the Higher Self of the person.

Fulcrums can also be verbal. A few well-placed words or phrases, relevant to the client's chosen Frame, or to what is happening in their body, can also help to facilitate change.

We evaluate, then place a fulcrum, pause, and then re-evaluate, careful not to overwork the body, using pauses to both amplify the effect and to give it time to process the work.

Note: In Acupuncture, needling a point can be seen as putting in a fulcrum for change. The needle introduces a clearer, stronger field at the site of the point, around which the energy of the point can reorganise, initiating change in the point and along its meridian pathway. Different needling techniques like twirling and thrusting add vectors to build the fulcrum.

WORKING SIGNS - Throughout a ZB session, the client will respond (or not) to the work and exhibit certain characteristic signs or spontaneous body signals indicating that the client is in a state of change, process or internal work (integrating energy and structure). Working Signs provide feedback to guide the practitioner in how best to proceed, or to pause.

Zero Balancing can give you a greater experience of your own body. My clients often say that Zero Balancing makes them more aware of their own body and their own energy. When I combine Zero Balancing with Acupuncture, my clients often tell me they can feel the energy going through their body and they accurately describe the meridian pathways to me.

Altered States of Consciousness

Fritz discovered that, during a Zero Balancing session, it was quite common for the client to go into altered states of consciousness normally achieved only by prolonged meditation, with clients also experiencing insights and ideas or inspiration to help the creative process:

"Touch can induce beneficial altered states of consciousness. It is a common goal in most meditative systems to 'quiet the monkey mind' in order to appreciate what lies beneath. This 'quiet mind' is actually an altered state of mind, different than our daily active thinking."
- Dr Fritz Smith

Altered or expanded states are also known as "non-ordinary states of consciousness", states of awareness outside the normal everyday, where new possibilities can emerge.

Fritz made two discoveries about touch:

1. The Left Brain (the linear, logical, analytical brain) is activated by input that comes in the form of a dot/dash system - like Morse code. This dot/dash input can be interrupted by holding constant pressure on the body, which leads to an expanded state of consciousness. This is particularly effective if the constant pressure is on bone.

2. When touching another person, there is a place, a moment, between one's in-push and out-pull, where the receiver will go into an altered state of consciousness. Specifically, if you press into a person's body with the same pressure that you are lifting off their body, the receiver will be unable to track you and they will go into an altered state.

So in the first instance a simple fulcrum of holding bone with constant pressure can lead to an expanded state of consciousness. And in the second instance a more complex fulcrum of doing two things at once can also have this effect. As Fritz says:

"If two apparently opposing stimuli are applied at the same time (for example pushing into the body with one hand while simultaneously pulling out with the other hand) then the Left Brain will be unable to keep track or make sense of both signals so it will go into an expanded state of consciousness or the Left Brain will go quiet."
- Dr Fritz Smith

In other words: When our Left Brain is confronted with the paradox of two complementary opposite sensations, held simultaneously, then our perception shifts to the Right Brain, which is the realm of intuition, creativity and imagination.

Hedonic ('hurt good)' fulcrums may invoke the paradox of simultaneous pleasure and pain. The mind can't hold it so it transcends out of the duality and into the experience of unity, and the client experiences the two as one. The hedonic level can take you away from your limiting beliefs, so that you discover and experience more of your true self.

"When a client is in an expanded state of consciousness they are less well held in their dysfunctional patterns and therefore more able to let go of them, to change and heal."
- Dr Fritz Smith

This suggests that healing and change is more possible in expanded states than in normal brain wave states.

Zero Balancing is like a working meditation for the practitioner. And it is so deeply relaxing that the client will often enter a meditative state and an expanded state of consciousness, encountering a stillness that exists beyond the thinking mind, where ideas and insights can 'bubble up' to the surface.

And I was to discover that, if a fulcrum is held for a longer period of time, then the client can sometimes have an inner journey experience. I share my own journey experience next:

My Journey

In May 2013 I qualified in Zero Balancing and a few weeks later I went on a 2-day Zero Balancing workshop on Physical Trauma Fields taught by Richard Walters in Devon. He led us in a guided meditation to connect to "The Stillness Field", shifting our awareness beyond the sounds we could hear. The idea was to put the Stillness Field in us, in our hands, and then to offer it to the other person.

I experienced The Stillness Field not as silence, as I expected, but as a 'Universal Hum'. This reminded me of Om - the original primordial Universal Sound that contains all sounds.

On the second day, we were working in pairs and I happened to be working with Richard. We finished the exercise before the rest of the group, leaving us with a few minutes spare. Richard invited me to lie down on the table again and simply said: "See what happens." Then he sat behind my head and did what felt like a Half Moon Vector at my neck, perhaps holding it for a little longer than I was used to, before taking his hands away and waiting...

I closed my eyes and immediately saw a winding green country road, which I followed, and as I engaged with it, the images became clearer in detail, and I soon came to a high, insurmountable brick wall. Then I noticed there was another wall, so that there was one on either side of me, corralling me onto a path. The path was clean, well lit by street lamps, clearly defined and signposted, leading up a hill in long gradual steps which had metal railings up the middle.

"If the path before you is clear, you're probably on someone else's."
- Joseph Campbell

This path was clear, defined, well maintained and structured, with an obvious direction. Despite this, I didn't particularly like it! I felt restricted and hemmed in by these high walls. And as soon as I acknowledged this to myself, I found myself "zooming out" and suddenly I was viewing this path from a gently bobbing boat safely out at sea. I wanted to stay there, preferring the calm freedom and expanse of the ocean to that strict regimented path.

However, as I relayed this to Richard, he encouraged me to explore further, so I returned to investigate the path. There was only one way to go, so I climbed the steps to the top of the path which led to a busy road full of speeding snarling traffic and honking horns. It didn't feel good, so I retreated and retraced my steps back down the path. Then I noticed there was now another path, this time leading downhill. It was dark, muddy and overgrown, perhaps even uninviting. It felt like few had gone here before, but I wanted to explore it, so I took this path and suddenly found myself traveling quickly. The momentum of going down the slope took me up the other side, and I felt so euphoric as I emerged effortlessly on an open hillside, wild and free in all directions, happy at last!

This inner journey felt important. It stayed with me and I needed to digest what had happened. Although I hadn't known what to expect, and the experience wasn't really framed except for a permissive "See what happens", in order to give my experience some context I noted that it occurred at a time when, having just qualified in Zero Balancing, I was wondering what was next and where my career would go from here. So, internally I had this question. To me the path I saw was a metaphor for my career path. Clearly something inside me did not want to follow the standard, clearly defined path with its restrictions. There were already plenty of people on that road, it didn't need anybody else joining in and doing more of the same. No, I wanted to explore where few others had, and the dark muddy path led me to freedom. And in exploring this work, which is the subject of this book, I have followed my own path - not always a clear path but ultimately the most rewarding, and it's the best thing I've ever done.

Exploring the Half Moon Vector (HMV) at the Neck

Naturally I was curious about what had happened. Richard later said he had put a fulcrum into my Higher Self (offering it to me at that level rather than working locally on my neck). I returned home to Brighton excited and eager to try this for myself to see if I could use the HMV at the neck to reproduce the kind of visual inner journey experience that I had just had in Devon, so that I could offer it to my clients. My first 'test pilot' was my friend Mike, whom I invited for a ZB session to try this out.

Toward the end of the ZB Protocol, just before the Closing Sequence, I used the following method:

- Pause to access the Stillness Field in myself, and bring this awareness into my hands
- Do an HMV (Neck) with the intention of putting the fulcrum into Mike's Higher Self
- Hold it... for longer than the usual 3-5 seconds, until I sense 'something happening' (while I keep focusing the Stillness Field into my hands)
- Finally disconnect, slide my hands out and wait for feedback

Success! Mike reported that a visual journey experience had begun as soon as I took my hands away - that's when it started. Buoyed by this we made several more attempts:

Mike "went to a different place" quite quickly, a dream place, like a lucid dream, and saw visual images, beautiful and positive: colours, shapes, spirals, and a book full of symbols. One time he opened his eyes and returned with tales of sea creatures of endless size emerging from water... Other times the experience was more physical, one of "standing where my own head was" and he experienced bodily sensations such as having extremely long arms... On another occasion he mentioned feeling an angelic presence, and peace.

Another volunteer, J.S., didn't experience images at first but a "flickering" and pleasant feelings of warmth, "like being inside a living, pulsing fire". Then she saw some drawings that she had done. When she went home and looked at her drawings, she realised that one of the pictures she had seen in the session was one she had drawn of her spirit guide.

In another attempt Mike got visual images but he suggested that I "do something at the feet". So I did an HMV at the feet and he reported that the experience opened up even more. Other times he said nothing happened until I did an HMV at the feet, as if this launched him. Later on other people reported that the HMV at the feet seemed to stop their experience! The HMV at the feet seemed to act as a switch, either starting and accelerating the visual experience, or stopping it completely. Usually it stopped the experience and brought the person back - perhaps it was distracting or perhaps touching the feet grounded the person.

Once, in a session with Mike, while I connected to the Stillness Field, I felt my heart opening and saw it fill with light which went into my hands (where my attention was) and Mike said he felt this energy, too! This happened spontaneously and unexpectedly and it felt important, so I decided to experiment with this "Heart Light" which had a stillness and constancy of its own. And it seemed to add power. So, as I applied the fulcrum, I imagined my heart opening and visualised the light beaming into my hands, offering it to the client.

That summer in 2013, I did several experimental sessions to try the HMV at the neck. However, despite some success and interesting results, as an Acupuncturist I also wanted to explore combining Acupuncture points with Zero Balancing, something Fritz had encouraged me to do in conversation a year earlier, in 2012, when I attended the annual Zero Balancing workshop at Gaunts House, Dorset.

I was particularly interested in finding Acupuncture points that might help to facilitate the same kind of visual inner journey experience that I had, while still hitching a ride on the altered states of consciousness that commonly occur in a ZB session. I felt that Acupuncture points may add an extra dimension or focus to the altered states while the physicality of Zero Balancing helps us to truly embody the experience.

What Are Acupuncture Points?

In Ancient Chinese philosophy humans are seen as existing "between Heaven and Earth". We are part of nature, which includes the cosmos, and we experience the influences of both Heaven and Earth. Heaven is the more subtle, unseen, energetic or Yang; Earth is more manifest, physical or Yin. Life is governed by the interplay of the Yin and the Yang within us, through the meridian system, which can be likened to a network of river channels which irrigate the terrain of our body. (To reflect this idea, I will call the meridians "channels".) At specific locations along the channel pathways we find the Acupuncture points.

So we are a microcosm, a miniature representation of the universe, within the macrocosm. The Acupuncture channels and their points facilitate communication between the inner microcosm and the outer macrocosm - between our body and our environment - and enable us to connect with deeper aspects of ourselves.

What we call Acupuncture 'points' are derived from the Chinese word meaning 'hole', or 'empty space', which implies access to the inner, and a hidden potential. We can enter the hole, the space, physically with an Acupuncture needle, or there are more esoteric practices for entering non-physically - entering the points with our mind in meditation.

The Ancient Chinese gave each of the Acupuncture points names to reflect their location, their function in the body, or their relationship between our inner and outer world. I believe the Chinese names of the Acupuncture points are important and many of them contain clues to what the points can actually do. Some of the names describe 'Gates' or 'Doors' to reinforce the idea that the points are portals between our inner world and the outer world.

To illustrate this, here is a practical example: One day while I was still training in Zero Balancing, one of my clients, Pamela, came to me for Acupuncture and I decided to work on her Lung channel. I was considering needling the point Zhong Fu, LU-1, in the hollow of the shoulder, but to save her undressing unnecessarily I decided to first do some Acupressure through her clothes and I began palpating along her Lung channel to check her response and see if it would be worth needling her there. Eventually I settled on the point Yun Men, LU-2, which is just under the collar bone, where it meets the shoulder. I touched this point on both sides. After a few minutes I stopped and went to feel her pulse. Pamela opened her eyes and said: "I felt as if I was flying through clouds!" (I had not told her that the point name Yun Men is translated into English as "Cloud Gate".)

Some people see Acupuncture points as buttons to press in order to change something in the body, or as a switch on a circuit to make something happen, but this view is simplistic. The Acupuncture points are alive. Like the rest of the body, they have a built-in intelligence - and they respond to consciousness. Acupuncture textbooks will list each point as having specific functions, which give clues to the point's potential, but these functions may require a certain context or technique. Whether or not we can access that potential and create the effect in clinic depends on where the client is at, also it depends on the practitioner. It is about creating the right conditions.

The point Yun Men, Cloud Gate, gave Pamela the experience of flying through clouds. Most textbooks attribute the point's name to its physical location (it is the highest point on the Lung channel and therefore nearest to the sky) or to the role of the Lung in the fluid metabolism in the physical body (the image of a rain cloud). Such physical explanations make sense but the Chinese name of an Acupuncture point can have a double meaning and refer to more than one thing simultaneously: not only on the level of the physical body but also on the level of the mind and spirit, as Pamela discovered.

Just as ZB fulcrums can be local or global, affecting different aspects or levels of a person, so it is for Acupuncture points. They provide us with possibilities but it depends on how we engage the point - the technique, the quality of touch, and the timing, among other things.

So began my exploration into the effects of using conscious touch on Acupuncture points, seeking inner journeys or visual waking dream experiences like the one I had in Devon.

Once again I enlisted the help of Mike to try out my ideas, and again my experiments were added onto the end of a Zero Balancing session in order to take advantage of the deep relaxation and expanded states of consciousness in ZB, making a positive response to the work more likely. So I was applying conscious touch to the Acupuncture points under these conditions, following a full ZB session.

Exploring the Effects of Conscious Touch on Acupuncture Points

I began drawing up a shortlist of likely Acupuncture points which might facilitate journeying in altered states, based on the points' functions, their nature, and their clinical applications. I focused especially on those points that are considered to have an effect on the mind and spirit of a person but that can also be located quickly and easily with the client lying on their back, fully clothed, so that the point(s) could be incorporated into the Zero Balancing Protocol.

I looked into the ancient Chinese names for the Acupuncture points - names that contain "Tian" (Heaven), "Shen" or "Ling" (words for Spirit), suggesting access to a higher state of consciousness, as well as names that include "Guan" or "Men" (Gate or Door), which on one level may refer to the physical passage of blood or fluids through the body but on another level suggest a portal to another realm, as previously revealed by Cloud Gate.

I considered Acupuncture points on the back which could perhaps fit seamlessly into the work we do on the back in Zero Balancing. There are points on the back with names like Soul Door and Spirit Door, which are used in Process Acupressure, a body/soul modality.

My method, echoing my HMV (Neck) experiments, was to access the Stillness Field in me, touch the points, put my mind in my fingers and offer the Stillness Field to Mike, with the intention of offering it to his Higher Self. With my fingers on the points, I would hold this clearer, stronger field for perhaps a minute, or until I sensed 'something happen'. Then I would take my fingers away, and wait for his feedback.

Zero Balancing is about touching the energy of bone, but most Acupuncture points are found in muscle or soft tissue, so I narrowed my search to those points located on bone. There are some points on the sternum but most of the points on bone are on the skull.

There are points on the skull that are associated with the mind and spirit. I selected points on the Bladder channel whose names hinted at possible interesting experiences: Cheng Guang, BL-6 ("Receiving The Light") and Tong Tian, BL-7 ("Heavenly Connection"), which are both located on top of the head and can be touched in combination together. They can elicit interesting responses but are not always easy to find quickly in thick hair.

There are some points on the Gall Bladder channel: Ben Shen, GB-13 ("Root of the Spirit"), and Toulinqi, GB-15 ("Head Above Tears"), which combine with Shen Ting, GV-24 ("Spirit Hall") on the Governing Vessel to form a row of five points inside the natural hairline on the forehead, known as the "Tiara Points", which can be used to calm a busy brain, although touching all five of them together (one midline, two either side) can feel awkward to hold.

The Governing Vessel is a channel running up the spine and over the midline of the head. There are some promising Acupuncture points here, in between the vertebrae of the spine. In one of my experimental sessions with Mike, sitting at the side of the massage table, I slid my hands under Mike's back to touch the vertebrae for the point Ming Men, GV-4 ("Gate of Life"), then tried two more 'spirit' points: Ling Tai, GV-10 ("Spirit Tower") and Shen Dao, GV-11 ("Spirit Path"). While I touched these last two points, Mike said his awareness moved from outside to inside his Third Eye, which corresponds to the point Yin Tang ("Hall of Impression") also on the Governing Vessel. So I sat behind Mike's head. With one hand under Mike's head to cradle his occiput, I used the index finger of my other hand to touch Yin Tang while imagining my Heart Light and focusing this light into my fingertip. Mike reported lots of abstract visual images while I gently held my finger there, but when I removed my finger the images disappeared, leaving him in a "dreamy space".

Again, similar to using an HMV at the feet, my finger on Yin Tang seemed to act as a switch, either generating images or stopping them completely just as we were getting somewhere. This seemed random and I found it puzzling and frustrating! So I stopped experimenting with Yin Tang, although I would later return to use it in order to encourage visual experiences, after seeing how it is used in other techniques to this effect. (See page 159)

Another point I tried was Tian Zong, SI-11 ("Heavenly Ancestor" or "Heavenly Gathering"), which is found on the shoulder blades. The name hinted at possible adventures and I wondered if Mike was about to experience a gathering of his heavenly ancestors. I sat at his head and slid my hands in flat under his shoulder blades, with my fingers on the points, holding with The Stillness Field and my Heart Light, before sliding my hands out again.

Mike said he had the experience of being very short, and in a different room to where we were, in which there was a surface, "like a liquid", and he was enjoying "dipping in and out of it". It was fun, "like a game of peek-a-boo". Then he watched as "several of me" took turns doing this, but "I wasn't the person, I was watching". It was as if they were children, which invoked feelings of warmth and compassion in him.

This may not be how I imagined a gathering of heavenly ancestors, although it did contain elements of connection and identification with others, and it was another exciting, interesting visual journey experience in an altered state.

Although I was looking for points that are located on bone, to be used with Zero Balancing, I couldn't help remembering Pamela's experience of "flying through clouds" while I touched Yun Men, LU-2 ("Cloud Gate"), which is in the soft tissue in the hollow of the shoulder, under the lateral end of the collar bone, and easy to find and add into the ZB Protocol.

So I decided to explore Cloud Gate further and, using the technique described in this book, more clients reported "flying through clouds" without any prompting. This particular point requires a very light, delicate touch to achieve this subtle effect, taking into consideration that the point itself can rise and fall with the client's breathing, which can affect the degree of touch.

Another point on soft tissue that called to me was Kun Lun, BL-60 ("Kun Lun Mountain"), which is behind the ankle joint, on the outside. It is related to the elements Fire and Water, and it is named after a mythical mountain in China that is significant in Taoist Alchemy.

So I tried this point on Mike, too. Sitting at the foot of the massage table I placed my index fingers on his Kun Lun points, touching them with the Stillness Field and my Heart Light, which did invoke some visual experiences. However, they were unremarkable until I decided to cradle Mike's heels in my palms as well, rather than just placing my fingers on the points. This felt more comfortable and supportive and Mike got visual images almost immediately, not a journey but more dreamy images coming and going, leaving him feeling very relaxed. Later Mike said he saw me as "a chameleon wearing clinic whites" (although I was not wearing my clinic whites on this occasion but a black T-shirt).

All of these points, when touched with the Stillness Field and my Heart Light towards the end of the Zero Balancing Protocol, resulted in some kind of interesting inner experience. I felt sure that they were not merely interesting but could also be useful to people in some way, as my own inner journey had been inspiring and useful in guiding me on my path.

I theorised that each Acupuncture point has a certain energy or quality that lends a certain influence or 'flavour' to the experience (what JR Worsley calls "The Spirit of the Point"). But I was also discovering that the experience depends on other factors, like the way the points are touched, how long to touch or hold the points for, and how long to wait after taking my hands away to allow the client time to respond.

I had experimented with many different points and naturally by now I had a few favourites, based on the experiences they had produced and the feedback Mike had given me. There were also practical considerations: some of the points were not always so easy to find quickly, and some points could feel awkward or uncomfortable for me to hold for too long. But my shortlist was getting shorter, and I was getting closer...

Window of Heaven Points

(Also Called "Window of the Sky" Points)

That summer I attended the annual ZB workshop at Gaunts House in Dorset. During a tea break I overheard some practitioners discussing altered states of consciousness and they mentioned Window of the Sky points (or Window of Heaven points) in Acupuncture.

The Window of Heaven points are a group of ten Acupuncture points which are considered to have a strong effect on a person's spirit. They are sometimes used to treat the person on a psychological and emotional level. The Window of Heaven points are as follows:

Tian Tu, CV-22, Heavenly Prominence
Ren Ying, ST-9, Person's Welcome
Fu Tu, LI-18, Support the Prominence
Tian Chuang, SI-16, Heavenly Window
Tian Rong, SI-17, Heavenly Appearance
Tian You, TH-16, Window of Heaven
Tian Zhu, BL-10, Heavenly Pillar
Feng Fu, GV-16, Wind Palace
Tian Fu, LU-3, Celestial Palace
Tian Chi, PC-1, Heavenly Pool

It should be noted that, although these ten points were listed together as a group in the ancient Chinese texts (Chapter 2 of the Ling Shu or "Spiritual Pivot"), they were not called "Window of Heaven" points; this name is a more recent addition. They were also not given any spiritual significance at that time. However, the Chinese names of most of these points contain the character Tian (meaning 'Heaven' or 'Sky'). In Chinese Medicine the term 'Heaven' can refer to the head, while the body is 'Earth'. Most of the Window of Heaven points are located on the neck - which is seen as the bridge between the head and the body - and they are used to regulate the ascending and descending flow of energy through the neck. (I wondered to what degree the HMV at the neck engages the Window of Heaven points.)

Because these points improve the flow of energy to the head, their use in Acupuncture treatments can have a strong psychological and emotional effect on the client, and this may have led to their use as spirit points.

The word 'window' evokes all sorts of images, suggesting opening a window of opportunity to a fresh new perspective, a skylight letting in light and clarity - allowing us to see things in a different way.

In Ancient China, Shangdi, the name of the Supreme Deity or God, was gradually replaced by the word "Tian" meaning Heaven or Sky. As a result, some references to Tian may in fact be veiled references to Shangdi, or God. So there is the idea that points with "Tian" in their name have spiritual significance or perhaps offer us access to the infinite mystery of the cosmos.

I wanted to combine Acupuncture points with Zero Balancing to explore altered states of consciousness, so I was looking for a point on bone that was easy to find and access within a Zero Balancing session (with the client fully clothed, lying on their back, face up) - a point that affects the mind or spirit. And since my own journey experience had been visual, I liked the idea of a point that also related to vision.

In Acupuncture theory there are Five Elements or 'Phases' of energy (like the seasons): Water, Wood, Fire, Earth and Metal. Each of these Elements is associated with specific organs and their channels and qualities. For example, the Wood Element is associated with the Liver and Gall Bladder, which are responsible for vision - physical, mental and spiritual vision - and it is also associated with the "Hun", that aspect of our spirit that relates to our imagination and dreams. The Hun is said to leave the body at night, free to journey to other realms.

So the Wood Element in particular seemed a likely one to use in my quest. In theory the Window of Heaven points had potential but they are all on soft tissue, not bone, and none of them belong to the Wood Element, so I appeared to be at a dead end.

The Acupuncture Point "Tian Chong", GB-9, "Penetrating Heaven"

One sunny day, on Sunday, July 21, 2013, I went for a walk in St Ann's Well Gardens in Hove, and decided to lie down on the grass in the sun. As I lay there thinking about Window of Heaven points, I suddenly remembered reading that a physician in the Ming dynasty, Ma Shi, had said that the point Tian Chong, GB-9 (Gall Bladder, Wood Element) should be listed as one of the ten points we know as the Windows of Heaven (instead of the point SI-17, Tian Rong). Tian Chong is translated into English as "Penetrating Heaven".

Tian Chong, GB-9, is the ninth point on the Gall Bladder channel. In Chinese Philosophy and the numerology of the I Ching, the number nine is considered a Heavenly number.

Giovanni Maciocia in "The Foundations of Chinese Medicine: A Comprehensive Text" states that the point, Tian Chong, GB-9, has "*a powerful mental effect*" and then goes on to say: *"It is interesting to note that, judging from the name and the indications, this point should be a Window of Heaven point but it is not mentioned as one. Its actions include two important actions of the Window of Heaven points: that is, subduing rebellious Qi from the head and calming the Mind."*

So here is a point, said to be a possible Window of Heaven, that has a strong effect on the mind, in the Wood Element (relating to vision), and it is on bone (the parietal bone just above the ear). What is more, it can fit nicely into the ZB Protocol and is easily accessible as I sit behind the client's head - perfect!

Most textbooks give the main indications for the point Tian Chong, GB-9, as headaches or tinnitus, but if that is all it is good for, I wondered why it is called "Penetrating Heaven". The Acupuncture points are multi-faceted and have the potential to work on many different levels; the effect depends on the context and conditions of the treatment, and how we engage the point.

I wondered if using Zero Balancing principles of touch on this specific Acupuncture point within a ZB session, while the client was in an expanded state of consciousness, could help the person to access the influences of Tian, or Heaven.

I had tried my technique on many different points and got interesting results and feedback with most of them, but switching from one point to a different point in the same session was sometimes intense and tiring for Mike, and I wanted to avoid overloading him by doing too much. I felt the need to limit the number of things I tried in a session, so rather than using several different points once each, it seemed better to choose one point and focus on that, visiting that one point several times in one session to explore it in more depth.

Tian Chong, GB-9, did indeed produce interesting experiences and feedback. In fact, the results were more promising than other points I tried. This point seemed to work better, in the sense that it consistently produced more interesting visual experiences or waking dreams, similar to my own journey.

In addition, it seemed significant that it had come to me in my daydream-meditation, as a natural bubble-up. It felt right. I settled on Tian Chong, GB-9, for simplicity, continuity and consistency. It is easy to locate, comfortable to hold, and it fits easily into the ZB Protocol. What is more, it is a (possible) Window of Heaven point; it is located on bone (on the skull); and it has a Wood Element flavour, which relates to vision.

By the end of 2013 I had decided to make Tian Chong, GB-9, my point of choice.

The Point Location (Illustration)

From "A Manual of Acupuncture" by Peter Deadman, Mazin Al-Khafaji with Kevin Baker:

(Note: A 'cun' is a measurement, roughly approximate to an inch or the width of the thumb)

Tian Chong, GB-9:
Above the ear, in the depression 0.5 cun posterior to GB-8, Shuaigu ("Leading Valley")

Shuaigu, GB-8:
In the temporal region, in the slight depression 1 cun directly above the apex of the ear

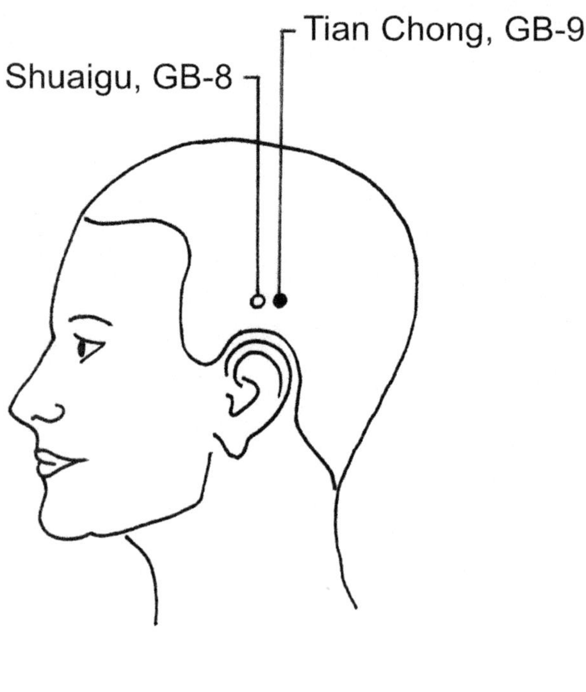

How to Find the Point Tian Chong, GB-9

(Note for non-Acupuncturists: you are not placing a tiny needle with precision, just a finger!)

To find the point, Tian Chong, GB-9, I place my index fingers just at the apex of the ears, then slide straight up to stop at a natural ridge or curve of the skull. My index fingers are now on the point Shuaigu, GB-8, approximately two finger-widths up from the apex of the ear. At first I would then slide my index fingers approximately one finger-width back, into the point Tian Chong, GB-9, directly above the posterior border of the auricle of the ear. Later, however, I found myself using my middle finger to touch Tian Chong, GB-9, partly because if I lay my hands flat at the sides of the client's head, with my fingers pointing down to the client's feet, then as my index finger moves up from the apex of the ear into position at Shuaigu, GB-8, my middle finger will naturally be in line with Tian Chong, GB-9, anyway.

(Like in most people, my middle finger is slightly longer than my index finger, so it will be just below the point. For this reason I need to bend it slightly so that it comes up level with my index finger.)

By coincidence, at the same time I was developing Penetrating Heaven, I was training in the Emmett Technique, a touch therapy developed by Ross Emmett which predominantly uses the middle finger, with other fingers tucked away to create more focus on the point. Inspired by this, with my fingers in the described position, I would then detach my index fingers from Shuaigu, GB-8, and tuck them away to leave the focus purely on my middle fingers on Tian Chong, GB-9.

Later on I had a dream that I was writing on a sheet of paper: "+ GB-8", and I knew it was about combining the two points Tian Chong, GB-9, with Shuaigu, GB-8, as a support point. (Sometimes in Acupuncture the point 'upstream' can act as a support to the next point. Interestingly, Yun Men, LU-2, Cloud Gate, is upstream from a Window of Heaven point, Tian Fu, LU-3, Celestial Palace.)

So sometimes I will leave my index fingers on Shuaigu, GB-8, with my middle fingers on Tian Chong, GB-9, and use both points in combination. This can feel more supportive to the client. Then, after a period of time on both points, I might detach my index fingers from Shuaigu, GB-8, and tuck them away to focus my middle fingers on Tian Chong, GB-9.

In short or fine hair it is easy to feel the bone and get a good bone-to-bone connection, but in thicker hair I tried to get in under the hairs to access and get in touch with the points - until I found that hair can serve as a 'buffer' to affect the level of touch, which is important. I will discuss levels of touch in more detail later.

When needling an Acupuncture point, the angle of insertion can determine the effect of the treatment, but with Penetrating Heaven I use my middle finger, Emmett style, perpendicular into the body.

Having made contact with the point, I then introduce a clearer, stronger field to the point. At first I used the Stillness Field. Later I tried a silent Om mantra, and I also explored visualizing my Heart Light, with my attention in my fingers on the points as my 'fulcrum'.

My idea for Penetrating Heaven was to apply the principles of touch from Zero Balancing to the point, Tian Chong, GB-9, which lies over the parietal bones of the skull. Although I am physically touching the client there, I am not working on the parietal bones physically; rather my focus is on the energy of the point, working on the level of mind (or Heaven).

Principles of Touch in Zero Balancing

Zero Balancing has a certain quality of touch. It is more than just physical touch or pressure. Part of the power of Zero Balancing is the quality of the touch at Interface. This is touch with clear boundaries, and with the attention of the practitioner (their mind awareness) in their hands.

INTERFACE - We touch at Interface: fully engaged but with clear boundaries of what is me and what is not; where I end, and where you begin. It means the client feels held in a safe, respectful way.

ATTENTION - In Zero Balancing we work with attention, not intention, i.e. simply noticing how it is, not wanting to change anything. "Feel what you feel", without judgement, comparison or preference.

So we don't just touch with our fingers but by putting our mind and attention in our fingers, making a bone-to-bone connection, working with our feeling mind, not our thinking mind. Touching with attention amplifies the effect.

Similarly, in Acupuncture, we can project our mind or awareness into the tip of the needle, and in my experience the results are more powerful when needled with attention and focus. In effect, we can extend these same principles of touch through the needle.

BLUE LINE - For Interface, we first need to 'take out the looseness' to get to the Blue Line, which is that certain point of tension or pressure that is sufficient to allow communication and feedback. (When I use Penetrating Heaven, because the point Tian Chong, GB-9, is on bone, there is not much looseness to take out, so I am already at the Blue Line. It doesn't require any pressure to access the point.)

NESTLE - The first touch is often to 'Nestle' or settle into the correct, comfortable position. Nestling invokes trust and support, already setting up the conditions for positive change.

PAUSE - After the Nestle there is a Pause, to prepare for the Fulcrum. So the 'formula' is in the following flow: Position (Nestle) - Pause - Action - Disconnect.

FULCRUM - The 'Action' is provided by the Fulcrum. Finger pressure, traction or rotation is used to create a specific field of tension, which is held constant for 3-5 seconds of stillness. (In Penetrating Heaven, however, the level of touch is lighter and I hold the points for longer.)

DISCONNECT - At the end of a Fulcrum we clearly disengage both energy and structure. The Disconnect is clear and distinct, to maintain the idea of boundaries and Interface.

(Note: When discussing Penetrating Heaven, I will break from ZB terminology and use the word "Release" instead of "Disconnect" to describe taking my fingers away from the point.)

After the Fulcrum follows another Pause to allow the client time to process the work and give a response. A Pause may be just a few seconds or as long as a minute or two.

My Penetrating Heaven technique originated directly from Zero Balancing but several other therapies have influenced my understanding of touch and are worth mentioning.

My Other Influences of Touch

Many touch therapies use a variation of the idea of working from the "Head, Heart and Hands". In ZB and in any bodywork it is not just about the practitioner being in their hands, but being fully in their body, rooted, grounded with their feet on the floor, regularly checking their own body for tension, constantly softening, relaxing and correcting their posture. This is particularly emphasised in Shiatsu, where the practitioner works from their Hara (or Dan Tien), the energy centre just below the navel.

Shiatsu

In my early years of exploring different therapies I did a short foundation course in Shiatsu, a Japanese bodywork that uses finger pressure on the Acupuncture points and channels.

One of the things I remember that influenced me from that training was the use of two hands: one Yin and one Yang, one 'listening', one acting. The "Mother Hand" holds the sacrum (or other site) in stillness while the "Working Hand" engages another site in action. Both hands are then used together, both listening and acting together as one, in tandem.

Sometimes an Acupuncture point may feel open, hollow and inviting. At other times it may feel closed, small, tight or tense, and reluctant to accept a finger (let alone a needle). In my Shiatsu training I learned that if a point feels closed or hard, then it is best to ease off and wait; if, on the other hand, a point feels open or soft, then it is better to engage further and go deeper.

Shiatsu was my first introduction to working with Acupuncture points. From there I went on to study Acupuncture at the International College of Oriental Medicine in East Grinstead.

Acupuncture

Acupuncture is more than just sticking needles in people. It also involves careful palpation. I was taught to locate the Acupuncture point with my finger and then spend a few moments palpating to prepare the Qi of the point so it is ready to meet the needle and respond.

This respectful approach is used in Zero Balancing as well. It is etiquette and good manners, like knocking at the door and waiting for permission to enter another person's territory.

Touch can give a sense of whether the Acupuncture point is open and receptive or not. It is as if the concept of the client's Donkey is present in the skin, so it is worth taking time to palpate in this way in order to prepare the point to receive the needle, giving the skin time to relax.

After inserting the needle into the surface of the skin you can pause, extend your sense of touch into the needle and, with your mind's attention in the tip of the needle, feel how far the point is willing to accept the needle, and if it is willing to allow you to insert it any further.

Most of the Acupuncture points are on both sides of the body and it is often interesting to touch the point on both sides simultaneously and compare them on the left and the right, sensing whether they feel different, or if you can feel a connection between the two points.

The Bowen Technique, developed by Tom Bowen

The Bowen Technique is a gentle therapy that works on the fascia (soft tissue). A typical move involves taking up the slack in the skin to engage with the underlying structure, offering a gentle held 'challenge' for a moment, then applying a rolling movement back over the muscle. Generally, the lighter the touch, the greater the effect.

The power of this gentle touch is shown by using a 50:50 mixture of cornstarch and water to represent the fascia of the body. If your fingers go in slowly and gently, then it allows you access and you can easily penetrate the surface. However, if you go in too hard or too fast, then it resists your finger. This phenomenon is also demonstrated in many internet videos of people adding cornstarch to swimming pools and then walking across the surface!

Bowen also uses the concept of the Therapeutic Pause, which involves typically waiting at least 2 minutes in between each set of moves in order to allow the body enough time to process the work.

The Emmett Technique, developed by Ross Emmett

The Emmett Technique is another therapy that uses gentle movements (or 'switches') over muscle, and it also uses finger touch to hold two points simultaneously until the first "jump" or response (working sign) occurs, after which there is a pause to allow the body time to process.

Emmett practitioners predominantly use their middle finger because it is more sensitive, and more balanced, as well as stronger and more direct, than any of the other fingers. The middle finger is applied perpendicular to the body. Any other fingers that are not being used are tucked away to create more focus and clarity of touch.

Less is More

All of these therapies adopt the principle of "less is more", both in the amount of work done and also in the amount of pressure used to do it. Each touch is like a message to the body.

Less work means that we avoid overloading the body with too many messages at once. 'More than enough' can be too much, like in the game "Don't Spill the Beans" where adding one more bean can make the whole thing collapse, wiping out the work that was done before.

Less work also allows us more time. The Therapeutic Pause gives the body enough time to process the work that we have done, and it allows something to happen in response.

It is not only the technique or the touch but also the pause that creates the desired effect!

Less pressure allows more to happen in response. Sometimes a gentle touch on the arm can be more comforting than a big bear hug. Similarly, if you speak in a soft, quiet voice, but with confidence, then people will pay more attention than they would if you make a big, loud noise.

As with a ZB "Donkey-lean", if you go in too quickly and forcefully or simply uninvited, then you meet with resistance. However, if you go in slowly and gently, the body will be more receptive.

We are giving a message to the body. If we deliver the message too forcefully, then it may be rejected. Force meets with resistance. And if we give the body too much information at once, then it can be confusing or overwhelming. Less work can have more of an effect.

Intention

Before we start journeying with Penetrating Heaven, I should talk about intention. In Zero Balancing we work with attention, not intention. There is intention in framing the session with the client but we use attention in our fulcrums, and pay attention to what happens, without any intention to make something happen.

We are not diagnosing and there is no judgement or comparison. We notice how the body is without wanting to change it, accepting it as it is. So there is no agenda. We are not trying to manipulate the body to be a certain way, and we are not trying to force anything to happen. We 'work with' rather than 'do to' the client, simply offering fulcrums as invitations or opportunities for change, with no attachment to the outcome. So the client has a choice.

Throughout my Zero Balancing training, creating altered states of consciousness was not seen as the primary goal; rather I would simply do the fulcrums and follow the Protocol, and the altered states would occur naturally as a by-product of the work, as Fritz had discovered:

"Since our body and our mind are one single entity, and they cannot be treated separately, every fulcrum will affect consciousness, so helping to create an expanded state for a client is not achieved by one particular fulcrum, it is a process that unfolds through the Protocol."

\- Dr Fritz Smith

The altered states are a product of the whole session; it is an accumulative effect of multiple fulcrums. The client is free to respond as they will and if the working signs indicate that they are in an expanded state, the practitioner may allow them more time so that they can make the most of the experience.

In Penetrating Heaven I hitch a ride on the back of the ZB Protocol to create conditions which make altered states of consciousness more likely. My idea was that the point, Tian Chong, GB-9, would add an extra focus or dimension, and perhaps allow the client to take things further.

A few months into my research, I attended a Zero Balancing workshop taught by Alan Hext entitled "The Structure of Energy" in which we discussed Zero Balancing and Acupuncture points. In my workshop notes I wrote down something Alan said:

"It can be seductive to think you can induce altered states of consciousness at will."

Indeed, yet here I was exploring how to induce altered states of consciousness by touch!

I quickly found that when it comes to clients experiencing altered states of consciousness, we can't make it happen. It is not something we can do on command. Even if the client is willing, there are many factors that can determine what happens and when.

The practitioner cannot have the intention to induce a particular altered state experience. However, in framing the session we can discuss the possibilities and wishes of the client, and the client can set their intention to *invite* an altered state experience. We can have the intention to create this possibility for the client and offer them the opportunity to have such an experience by creating the right conditions where altered states are more likely and facilitate the experience, if the client is willing, by working with them and their intention.

The Frame contains the client's intention for the session. The Frame will help to focus and influence what happens. It can also provide a reference or context to help us understand what happens for the client in the session.

So, in Penetrating Heaven I am not imposing, but simply offering. I am putting a clearer, stronger field in myself. Then I put my awareness in my hands, my fingers on the points, and offer this field to the client as an invitation or opportunity to explore possibilities. That's all we *can* do.

Early Trials of Tian Chong, GB-9, Penetrating Heaven

Initially I lacked confidence in whether Penetrating Heaven would really work. I assumed it would be necessary to do Zero Balancing first for the client to access an expanded state of consciousness. So I would do the Zero Balancing Protocol and add my Penetrating Heaven technique on at the end. If it didn't work, then at least the client would get a good ZB session out of it!

In Zero Balancing, a fulcrum introduces a clearer, stronger field - an unwavering constancy which is held in stillness. It is around this Still Point that the energy has an opportunity to re-organize, and change.

My method, as before, was to access the Stillness Field in me, then touch the points, Tian Chong, GB-9, equally on both sides, put my mind in my fingers and offer the Stillness Field to the client, with the intention of offering it to their Higher Self. Holding the points, I would hold this clearer, stronger field for perhaps a minute, or until I sensed 'something happen'. Then I would take my fingers away, and wait for feedback.

(I considered alternating my touch on the points, from one side to the other, using two opposing stimuli at the same time to encourage an expanded state of consciousness. However, this was not necessary. Simply holding the points equally on both sides with the Stillness Field was enough.)

I had experienced the Stillness Field as Om, the Universal Sound, and in time I gradually started to use a silent Om mantra as my still focus while touching the points in this way.

I had also had the experience of feeling my heart opening and being filled with light, which also had a stillness and constancy. This led me to try using my Heart Light as my focus when I touched the points, imagining my heart being open and visualizing the light in my heart flowing into my hands, offering it to the points. This often made the client's experience more visual.

From my Acupuncture training I knew that the heart is likened to the emperor of the body. In Ancient China the Emperor was considered to be the embodiment of Heaven, ruling with clarity and wisdom. So the heart's role is to be a void (i.e. clear and uncluttered, in calm stillness), that it may receive the influences of Heaven. Therefore, Heaven is 'up there' but it is also within us, in our heart.

We experience Heaven through our heart, which would suggest that it is good for us to consciously drop down out of our head and into our heart, and place our awareness there. I saw it as my Heart Light (my 'Heaven') connecting with the client's Window of Heaven, and later on I would experiment with the idea of actively bringing light down from Heaven.

These were the different methods I used to introduce a clearer, stronger field to the points: The Stillness Field, a silent Om mantra, and my Heart Light. I would usually choose one, or sometimes combine them, for example, using the silent Om to back up my Heart Light.

To summarise, my 'technique' at this early stage was to begin with a pause, settle myself, feel my feet on the floor and my body on the chair, and take some slow, deep breaths to centre myself. Then I would locate the points, and touch, nestle and pause to put my mind in my fingers. Next, I would offer my clearer, stronger field: either in the form of the Stillness Field, a silent Om, or my Heart Light. I would hold this constancy until I sensed something happen, then take my hands away and pause, allowing enough time for the work to take effect, and wait for feedback. Then I would repeat my technique for another attempt, or, as I called it, a 'Run'.

A word on the term 'Run': Originally, I called each attempt a 'Journey' because that described my own experience, and I hoped that a similar thing would happen for my clients. However, not everyone had a journey experience every time. Many clients did journey during a session but it sometimes required more than one attempt before this happened, so I use the term "Run" to refer to each time I touch the points, apply my technique, and take my hands away for a pause. Typically, I would do my technique three times at the end of a ZB session, making it a total of three Runs.

To give a fuller picture of how I worked in those early days, and how and why Penetrating Heaven developed the way it did, I will now present a snapshot of those early sessions.

In the early experimental stage, the Frame for the session was simply: "See what happens!" This was a journey into the unknown, and I was learning as I went along.

In the first trial session of Penetrating Heaven, I touched the points and held them. Before I had even let go, Mike had the experience of floating up out of his body. However, he felt that my touch was too heavy and intrusive ("Like pressing buttons"), and as he floated up out of his body, his head remained anchored by my fingers so that he couldn't take off properly and was left floating upside down. Mike felt sure that if I had taken my hands away at the right time, he would have flown off and enjoyed an astral travel journey.

It was an early lesson that the key to this subtle work is a lighter touch, and timing!

Generally, when I touched the points, Mike would start to see "lots of images" even though he had not had any visuals prior to me touching these points during the Zero Balancing work. Sometimes his visual experience would consist of 'random' images, lights, geometric shapes, swirling patterns or symbols. Once he saw a flower, which then appeared out of his chest with a feeling of openness, so he did not merely receive images but also feelings to go with them. As we settled into a familiar routine, later attempts gave Mike a fuller journey experience:

"I emerged in space, feeling comfortable and gently floating. I floated down to earth but the ground I walked on was the inside of a hollow cylinder that I could walk around and around forever. I soon became bored of this material world and flew off. As soon as I did, space opened up to another reality beyond. Here, I was in a spiritual realm and saw before me a gold object: 3 gold spheres linked by a triangle of concave, gold strips. Though apparently metal, this object moved towards me and I absorbed it. Another identical object appeared before me, which I also

absorbed. This happened many times. I felt energised by receiving these until I became a large version of the object myself."

And, in another session:

"I entered a red space but felt that I was unable to go further. I think some tension in repressing fatigue was why. For the second journey [Run] I was ready and experienced waves of bliss as in deep trance or transcendence and saw the events and aspirations of my life all laid out around me and progressing with ease. I then fell deeper and perhaps lost awareness here and there but had a sense of healing being sent to a friend in the form of the red space I had experienced previously surrounding him. I had not been thinking about him and am not consciously aware that he is in need of healing."

Gaining more confidence, I offered my Penetrating Heaven technique to more people: Claire reported seeing colours. Then she saw a keyhole but wasn't able to go beyond it. A light went over her head but she couldn't follow it. I wondered if she might get the key next time! In her next session she saw "a square box of brilliant white light" and a similar feeling to the keyhole of light in the previous session, and again, she couldn't go through it.

In another session Claire set a frame for more focus in her divorce proceedings. She floated up, and saw herself lying on the massage table with me sitting behind her. She saw herself cutting red strings that were binding her or holding her. She was doing this from above herself. She also said that her heart expanded and opened up, and there was "lots of white light". In the days after the session, she reported that she had felt stronger, "more fierce", in dealing with her ex-husband, and that she stood firm in her settlement.

Working Signs: Early Responses

At first I would close my eyes while I was touching the points to help me to concentrate, as I was earnestly trying to do it right. But eventually I progressed to doing it with my eyes open, so that I could actually observe the client!

It wasn't always obvious that something was happening. But I relied on the Working Signs that serve as a feedback loop in Zero Balancing to monitor the client's response. These are certain characteristic signs or spontaneous body signals indicating that the client is in a state of processing or internal work.

"A working sign means something significant is happening, or just happened, to the client."
- Dr Fritz Smith

Working signs relate to both the energy body and the structural body, and are reflected in both of these bodies:

"When the vibratory field of the energy body shifts, becoming more harmonic with the structural body, then this shift from one vibration to another stimulates a working sign."
- Dr Fritz Smith

The first obvious Working Signs to notice are the client's breathing and eye movements:

BREATHING - There may be changes in the speed and depth, or in the rhythm of the breathing. Sometimes the breathing will seem to go through a brief 'excited' phase where it is quicker and busier, like something is happening, or as if the client is processing. Other times the breathing will be more of a relaxed flow, and it may seem very deep and slow. It can also be preoccupied or hesitant, as if the client is working things out.

THE WORKING BREATH CYCLE - During Zero Balancing the client can go into a state of deep relaxation, so their body has little demand for oxygen. As a result, their normal breathing pattern will move into no breath or a very shallow breath for a period of time, followed by a big deep involuntary breath and a return to normal again.

EYE MOVEMENTS - There may be eye flutters or movement side to side, as if the client is 'searching'. However, I learned that rapid eye flutters do not necessarily indicate a visual experience.

FACE - The client's facial expression can give clues as to what is going on, and sometimes the client's demeanour may change or their features may look different.

OTHER WORKING SIGNS:
Kriya - Spontaneous twitches or movements of the body, resulting from a shift in energy.
Swallowing - This may indicate emotional processing, or coming out of a deeper state.
Borborygmi - The gurgling of the intestines as a result of parasympathetic nervous system activity while the body is at rest and going into deeper states of relaxation.
An increase in pulse - This can be palpable or sometimes visible, also signifying activity.

Sometimes the environment reflects working signs and the room may suddenly go quiet.

Remember that Zero Balancing is an invitation to change, i.e. the practitioner can't make change happen. But the client can stop it happening, and sometimes there appears to be no response. So it is useful to know that:

"There is no such thing as no response,
because even no response is still a response."
- Dr Fritz Smith

Responses to Penetrating Heaven

When I was doing case studies for my certification in Zero Balancing, one of my clients showed little sign of what she was about to feed back. As she lay on my massage table, I didn't see any obvious working signs and I assumed the session wasn't going very well. However, when we finished, she sat up, smiled, and told me she had been back at her father's death bed with him, having the conversation that she wished she had had when he died the previous year. This was a lesson to me that, even though it may look as if nothing is happening, everyone is having their experience.

And it was the same with Penetrating Heaven. The client would not necessarily show working signs all the time, and after I took my hands away for a couple of minutes, it seemed a long time to wait for feedback, so I felt relieved when my client confirmed something was happening.

Types of Responses

Because my own journey experience had been visual, I had looked for Acupuncture points that I thought might help to facilitate visual experiences, so I was expecting Penetrating Heaven to give people visual experiences similar to the one I had.

Most of Mike's early experiences were indeed very visual but occasionally they were more of a body-felt experience. One time he said he initially felt as if he was bending out of his body, "exploring", then he felt as if his body was arching, with the sensation of being elsewhere, "in a spiritual place". I did not observe Mike's body physically arching, although I have since witnessed this in other clients as they displayed quite dramatic kriya.

Another early volunteer, J.S., had purely non-visual experiences. She said she had the sensation of feeling something inflatable over her stomach and torso - not a negative feeling but "curious". She also felt as if her head was moving gently from side to side, then a feeling of rocking from side to side "as though I'm a round object on a hard floor". At one stage I noticed her frowning and looking puzzled. This corresponded to her feeling as if someone had just presented her with a big fish and placed it in both her hands, which surprised her. The fish was “difficult to hold, and heavy”.

As I did more sessions with different people, I learned that, although most people do get images (visual sense), some people are more attuned to movement and/or feelings (kinesthetic sense), or to listening (auditory sense), or even to smelling/tasting (olfactory/gustatory sense) - but most people did get something!

It would be a mistake, however, to label people as ‘visual’ or ‘kinesthetic’, for example, because some ‘non-visual’ people still reported seeing colours and images, and alongside these they got words or feelings, too. Some people may start with a non-visual experience and only get words or feelings, and then in a later session they start to get images as well. Other people would get visual images for the first sessions but in later sessions they would only receive words (that were meaningful to them), and so I prefer to think that there are not ‘types’ of people but types of responses.

Clients often tell me that their experience ”is not in real time” and that the expanded states are “beyond the duality of time and space”, and for this reason they can lose track of time. A five-minute Run can feel like an hour, meaning that an hour-long session can feel like they have been gone a very long time.

Developing My Touch

As I offered Penetrating Heaven to more people and received a wider range of feedback, a number of common key elements emerged that seemed important to the process.

A Light Touch (Less is More)

In the early trials of Penetrating Heaven my main focus had been on the Stillness Field rather than on a specific level of touch, so I was simply placing my fingers on the points, with a good bone-to-bone connection. And although I didn't intend to apply any pressure, Mike's experience of floating up out of his body but being anchored by my fingers showed that my touch had been a bit heavy and too physical at first. I had also held the points for too long when I should have released and taken my fingers away to allow him to float off.

This led to a greater appreciation of the importance of a light touch and the correct timing, i.e. how long to hold, when to release the points, and how long to wait to allow the Run enough time to take effect.

Although altered states of consciousness can still occur with a firm touch, if my touch was too heavy it seemed to inhibit the client's experience. It was as if we were trying to drive with the brakes on. Less is more - a lighter touch allows more to happen.

Sometimes my technique produced uninhibited journeys before I fully released the points, but client feedback suggested that this was when I had used a touch that was lighter than usual.

So I began to consciously develop a lighter touch, still physically touching the points so the client can feel my fingers there, but lighter, which also calls for more focused attention. And it was during a regular ZB swap session where I was working with a lighter touch that my friend Mandy reminded me of the importance of attention, which really is key to this work.

Charge Me Up and Let Me Go! - "Nothing Happens Until You Take Your Hands Away"

When I explored the HMV (Neck), I would hold the fulcrum for a certain time, then release and wait. Similarly in Penetrating Heaven, many clients told me that, while I was holding the points, my fingers seemed to "charge them up", ready to go. (One client described it as "like telephones connecting".) But things only really started to happen when I let go and took my fingers away. Most clients agreed: "Nothing happens until you take your hands away."

"The Release Seems Important"

But it was more than simply taking my hands away. In feedback, Mike specifically told me: "The release seems important." Until then I had not been paying particular attention to how I released the points - it was more like just 'removing' my fingers, and perhaps too abruptly sometimes, in a rather crude "touch, hold and release" mechanism. But now, as I began to practice a lighter touch, more clients reported that things started to happen while I was still touching the points, so I decided that I would take my fingers away much more gradually in a slow, mindful release so as not to disturb the client's experience.

The Release is indeed important, not only how long to hold, but also when to release and how to release (slow and gradual works best). This revealed that another key element of touch is timing, including the pacing and pauses that we use in Zero Balancing (see later).

(Note: When discussing Penetrating Heaven I will break from ZB terminology and use the word "Release" instead of "Disconnect" to describe taking my fingers away from the points. This is simply because "Release" was the term that Mike and I used in our discussions.)

Secrets of the Skull

Back in 2012, while I was still on my way to becoming a certified Zero Balancer, I attended a workshop taught by Judith Sullivan and Mary Murphy called "Secrets of the Skull". It focused on how to apply the principles of Zero Balancing to the bones of the skull, and how they can be used to affect the structures within the skull, including some fulcrums for the brain.

Judith and Mary both have a background in Cranio-Sacral Therapy, and their approach added a different dimension for me, further expanding my appreciation of mindful touch. And because I was working with the point Tian Chong, GB-9, which is located on the parietal bones of the skull, this workshop was to be an important influence on my Penetrating Heaven technique.

As I continued my research into altered states of consciousness I found myself exploring how different brainwave states are involved in the resulting inner journey experiences and how each lobe of our brain relates to different sensory perceptions and types of response.

During the Brighton Festival in May 2014, Mike told me that there was an art exhibition on the theme of Dream Imagery. In it, the artist David Nicholls displayed some work depicting his experiences in dream state and out-of-the-body experiences.

I went along and the first picture I happened to see was called "Joined at the Head" which reminded me of Mike's feedback from his first trial session of Penetrating Heaven. The image showed the astral body floating above the body on the bed, except that it was still rooted to the head as the rest of the body floated up, leaving him upside down.

The artist, David Nicholls, introduced himself and I told him about my work. He mentioned another festival event that was happening that week, a lecture on Lucid Dreaming by Luciana Haill and Sarah Janes.

At the Lucid Dreaming lecture, we were shown feedback from an EEG (Electroencephalogram), measuring the brainwaves during lucid dreams. This gave me the idea to measure brainwaves during a Penetrating Heaven session. Although my own research didn't get off the ground, I'm pleased to hear that such research into Zero Balancing is being conducted in the USA. The Zero Balancing Touch Foundation (ZBTF) has teamed up with the Neuro Synchrony Institute in Austin, Texas, using an EEG to measure brain wave activity during a ZB session.

"Early results for brain activity during Zero Balancing sessions suggest ZB Touch may facilitate a deep change in brain patterns [expanded states of consciousness] more widely associated with the benefits of meditation."
- The Zero Balancing Touch Foundation (ZBTF)

The Lucid Dreaming lecture inspired me to revisit what I had learned in the Secrets of the Skull workshop, and I experimented with the brain fulcrums to enhance the effects of Penetrating Heaven.

Although the brain fulcrums were helpful, I was wary of doing too much and overloading the client, so after a while I decided that the brain fulcrums should be kept in reserve, as an option for when the client feels that nothing is happening, which I will discuss later.

The important thing was that Secrets of the Skull helped me to develop my touch. And just a few months later, in October 2014, I went to a Skull Review Day with Judith in London, which was very timely as I was still perfecting my Penetrating Heaven technique then.

Principles of Touch on the Skull

The Secrets of the Skull workshop introduced me to a lighter touch than I was used to, and I also learned to hold fulcrums for longer than the standard 3-5 seconds while still remaining fully present at Interface. This is important in Penetrating Heaven.

Because the skin and soft tissue on the skull are thin, there is not much looseness to take out, which means when you touch the skull you are very quickly at the Blue Line (where communication begins) and your fingers can make a good bone-to-bone connection easily.

As a result, we use a lighter touch which is more about the energy than the structure - touch with attention. Also, we hold fulcrums for longer in an approach that I remember as "Hold, Listen and Allow".

In Zero Balancing we use our feeling mind, not our thinking mind: "Just feel what you feel." We touch the bone, sensing or 'listening' with attention while we hold our awareness in our hands, and meet what is there without judgement or comparison, simply noticing how things are.

"If you can balance something to neutral without judgement or comparison by holding it in its own space, it will naturally move to its highest possible benefit."
- Dr Fritz Smith

It is as if by meeting things in the moment exactly as they are, our witnessing in this way is reflected back to the body, helping it to know itself and orient itself, so it can find a way home again. If we acknowledge how things are, the act of simply being present with them can invite them to change.

When working on the skull, we hold the fulcrums for a longer time. But first we begin with a respectful approach, as if knocking at the door, waiting for a response, requesting permission to enter. So you introduce yourself before you introduce the clearer, stronger field - and the clearer, stronger field in this case is less about holding with physical pressure and more about holding with attention.

Having made a good bone-to-bone connection, we then start to gradually ease off into a lighter touch while still maintaining meaningful contact and connection. And because our touch is lighter, we can more easily and comfortably hold the fulcrum for a longer time.

A lighter touch gives 'breathing' space and leaves some room for the point to 'work'. It allows movement, communication and energy (or information) to flow under my fingers. As an analogy we can think of a boat in a harbour that is not tied too tightly to its mooring but is given some 'wriggle room', some freedom to move with the flow of the water.

The art is feeling how light you can be, how much you can ease off, and still be present. Therefore, a lighter touch means you have to pay even more attention to what you are feeling.

Touch with less pressure allows more to happen - it allows more energy flow, more information flow. Touch with less pressure also means we pay more attention, so we can feel more of what is happening.

This was exciting. I was discovering the importance of a light touch that is held for longer, with a slow, mindful release. Doing everything slowly increases our attention, and our attention amplifies the effect.

Touch with attention is key. Therefore, if you notice your mind wandering, or if you get distracted or bored, then it is time to stop. Take your hands away and start again, or finish and move on.

Conscious Touch With Attention (Hold, Listen, Allow)

ZB is a working meditation, with an emphasis on attention. You are in the present moment, exactly as it is - not as you think it should be, and not wanting it to be different - with your mind in your hands. You meet the person there, at Interface, and you "Hold, Listen, and Allow".

Hold

'Hold' means to maintain a certain quality of touch at Interface, to meet the client with consistent support, and to hold the stillness in constancy. Holding for longer requires a lighter touch, so that the hold can be sustained comfortably.

Holding for longer also requires us to be mindful of maintaining Interface with attention. In other words, we hold physically but we also hold with attention and awareness, and this needs to be sustained.

Listen

'Listen' means to pay attention to, not just with our ears but with all our senses. It means to perceive what is there, or what may be happening, so that we may receive this information and witness it. Listen with an innocent curiosity. Listen like anything is possible - you may learn something!

To be a good listener, you spend time listening to what the other person is expressing so that you can understand how things are for them. You don't assume that you already know what is happening, merely waiting for your turn to add your own input.

In order to listen, we need to allow the other person to express, so ease off the finger pressure and use a lighter touch so that you don't smother or suffocate the point - it is trying to talk to you! A lighter touch, like a softer voice, requires more attention so that you can really sense what is going on.

Therefore, be in your hands. Put your attention in your fingers on the point and really listen: What does the point have to 'say'? What is happening under your fingers? Sometimes it may feel as if the point is 'breathing', or there may be a pulsing movement, or a rhythm like a wave. Sometimes it may feel alive with activity. Feel its dance and know that the body is alive. Wherever we touch someone, there is a lot going on there, in every cell. I find it useful to remember that the dance of 'The 10,000 Things' is going on right now under my fingers if I will only put my attention there and listen for it - and suddenly I will feel something! Imagine that every cell of the body contains a consciousness, an intelligence, even a personality, and listen...

"Everything speaks if you know how to listen."
- Jason Kirkey

Allow

'Allow' means to feel what you feel and let it be, accepting it as it is in the present moment. Notice without judgement, without assuming you know how it should be, without making it wrong or trying to fix it, without wanting it to be any different - allow it to be and to express, but equally allow it to change if it wants to, when it wants to and in the way that it wants to.

Again, this requires a lighter touch, easing off the finger pressure to allow the point the necessary 'breathing' space, allowing free movement and expression, allowing whatever happens to happen. And allowing requires a lighter attitude - get out of the way mentally. Surrender your agenda in order to create space for something to happen and so that you have 'something' to listen to.

Just be there as a quiet presence, as an open mind with no agenda except 'This is what I am doing':

I touch with attention, with my mind in my fingertips, and I simply Hold, Listen and Allow it to be. I *Hold* the stillness, *Listen* and pay attention, and *Allow* things to be as they are, or to change as they will.

The Power of the Pause

I have already introduced the idea of the Pause in Zero Balancing: We pause before we take action, to prepare for something to happen; and we pause after taking action to allow something to happen. There can also be pauses within a fulcrum: We pause when we get to the Blue Line, and we pause before we add another vector when building a fulcrum.

"In Zero Balancing we use the pause as a working tool.
It's different to a stop. You haven't let go, there's still tension.
It's a pregnant pause, you are still holding the field."
- Dr Fritz Smith

Similarly, a public speaker or comedian will pause for effect during their monologue in order to build the tension... and then pause for effect after delivering their verbal fulcrum (or punchline).

There is power in the pause. The pauses are just as important as the work, and they help to create the overall effect. The pause allows time for the client's response and enables the person to reap the full benefit from the work.

As in music, where the pause in between the notes and the tempo of the piece create the effect, we do not try to force things by doing too much, and we do not try to force the pace, either. We use a gentle touch and a gentle pace, with pauses to allow the body enough time to respond.

"The body appears to naturally, spontaneously demand pauses
in the therapeutic process."
- Louise Tremblay, The Therapeutic Pause

The idea of the Therapeutic Pause has also been adopted by other bodywork therapies. The Bowen Technique, for example, requires a wait of at least 2 minutes in between each set of moves in order to allow the body enough time to process the work and its effect.

In Zero Balancing, the pauses may last just a few seconds or as long as a minute or two. I had already experimented with borrowing the 2-minute pause from Bowen and inserting it in between key stages of the core Zero Balancing Protocol (specifically, after working on the lower back, after the hip fulcrum, and after the HMV at the feet) and I found that by offering longer pauses clients seemed to enjoy deeper expanded states of consciousness.

Now, for my Penetrating Heaven technique, I was learning how long I should pause for each Run in order to give the client enough time and opportunity for a response at a deeper level.

The book Sabbath by Wayne Muller explores the concept of how, in religious traditions, a Sabbath is a pause for rest. A Sabbath means to stop work, which gives other things space to happen naturally and allows deeper things to come to the surface. Muller also talks of the idea of 'being sabbath' for someone else, so the pause is not just a length of time, but time held in the present moment with someone as a witness.

"Sometimes it's necessary to stop one thing
before another thing can begin."
- Wayne Muller, Sabbath

Farmers know that, when a field is left to rest and lie fallow for a while and given a pause from the relentless cattle hooves or ploughing work, it allows previously dormant seeds the opportunity to flourish in "the sweet soil of time" so that 'new' varieties of herbs and flowers can now appear which were unknown there during times of working activity.

Likewise, seeds in our mind can sprout and come up during the pauses in Zero Balancing, and deeper parts of us have an opportunity to grow. The pause allows our fruit to ripen.

The Art of Timing

From the earliest experimental sessions it became clear that, as well as a certain quality and lightness of touch, there was another key factor to consider - the length of time that each stage requires:

I need to hold the points for a long enough time to 'charge them up' before I release them, but not hold for too long in case it inhibits the effect. I need to release at just the right time. Then I need to pause and wait for a long enough time after the Release in order to allow the Run to fully take effect and to harness the power of the pause.

How long to hold my fingers on the points to 'charge them up' before I release

I didn't accurately measure the length of time that I held the points because keeping time while concentrating on my technique was distracting. But I began by touching the points for about a minute or so, applying my technique, then taking my hands away to allow enough time for the client to have their inner journey experience. (Early feedback had suggested that nothing happened until I took my hands away.)

Later on, as I adopted a lighter touch, I would hold the points for longer - several minutes - including the time to nestle into the points, ease off, apply my technique and detach slowly and gradually. (Later feedback had suggested that a lighter touch, and a longer, slower, gradual Release, are important.)

Eventually, with practice and experience, the timing - how long to hold the points, and how long to wait after the Release - became intuitive and I was guided by the working signs. A note in my journal: "Put your mind in your fingers at all times, sense when to come off."

How long to wait after the Release to allow enough time for the Run to take effect

To decide how much time to wait for a Run to take effect, I was influenced by my training in the Bowen Technique, which requires that we wait at least 2 minutes in between each set of moves in order to allow the client's body enough time to process the work. So, in the beginning I decided to insert a pause of 2 minutes after I released the points.

After a pause of 2 minutes I would check in with the client and ask what was happening. Sometimes their experience had started almost immediately and was now well underway; other times it could take the full 2 minutes just to begin to happen. One client, who had had immediate responses in previous sessions, told me: "Sometimes it takes time to work."

Experience showed that, if something is going to happen, then it will have started within 2 minutes of me taking my fingers off the points.

As I have said, although the inner experience can start immediately when I release (or even while I'm still touching), sometimes it will need the full 2 minutes just to get going. And so I would wait patiently for a whole 2 minutes before checking in with the client, only to be told with mild annoyance that I had interrupted them just as it was getting good! In such cases we would simply try again and make the next Run a few minutes longer than before.

I found that usually (but not always) a Run of 2 minutes is too short to be fully satisfactory, meaning that it is not enough time for the client to fully engage with their experience. However, it is enough time to gauge the client's response, so I continued to use 2 minutes for the first Run to 'test the water' and to confirm that the process had begun to happen.

And then, if it was going well, I increased the second Run to 5 minutes, and gave them whatever time was remaining for a third and final Run, which was often up to 10 minutes.

(Note: When I talk about the length of a Run, I am referring to the length of the Pause after I take my hands away and complete the Release. So these are pauses of a full 2, 5 and 10 minutes each.)

Most of my sessions took place in a clinic room rented by the hour, so I had enough time to do the Zero Balancing Protocol (20-40 minutes) and then add Penetrating Heaven at the end. This meant that usually there was enough time in the session for me to repeat three Runs of increasing length.

I assumed that each Run would take the client progressively deeper, and that as they went deeper, they would need longer to have their experience. And so it evolved into three Runs, each one longer than the one before. Typically, I started with a 2-minute Run as an introduction to check the client's response, followed by a 5-minute Run, and then finally a 10-minute Run. This left enough time at the end of the session for the client to come back down to earth and share feedback.

I liked the idea of having three attempts, or Runs, as this fitted nicely into an hour-long session. It also relieves the pressure to get a result straightaway because we get more than one shot at it.

The first Run serves as an introduction to test the water, so both the client and the practitioner know what to expect, like a warm-up or practice run. Then the second Run allows the client more time to explore their inner experience. And finally, the third Run gives them an opportunity to revisit their journey or to explore it more deeply, building to a grand finale.

The client's experience could therefore progress in three gradual steps, with a beginning, a middle and an end, with pauses in between to allow me to check in and get feedback from them.

And three Runs seemed to be enough. Even in experimental sessions at home, when I had all afternoon to work with a friend, the third Run still seemed to be a natural limit because any further attempts (Runs) after that resulted in the experience tailing off and reaching a plateau.

In the early stages, in my eagerness to get feedback, I would often check in with the client too soon, which then made me reluctant to interrupt them for fear of ruining their experience. However, this was never really a problem. On one occasion I did interrupt an experience too soon, just as the client was starting to receive images. But to my surprise I heard myself say: “Don’t worry, I can take you back there.” Then I simply repeated my Penetrating Heaven technique, and it did indeed take them back to where they had left off.

Feedback confirmed that people have more of an experience if I give the Run more time - or rather, if I give the Pause more time. An essential ingredient in each Run is the long pause which allows things to happen and to fully take effect. The Pause - that period of stillness where I don’t do anything - is where the magic happens!

In the end I found that a good Run needs to be at least 5 minutes long; although 10 minutes is even better. It felt a long time to wait for feedback yet most clients told me that they wanted more time! In one memorable session I had allowed the final Run a good 10 minutes and was about to bring the session to a close but there was still time, so I held off for a few minutes more. After the session the client told me that in those few extra minutes she had moved into a deeper state and had a profound experience that would otherwise not have happened.

So, in cases where working signs are obvious and abundant, when I am confident my client is having a good experience, I let them go on for longer. Of course, at this stage of developing my technique, as I was adding all three Runs onto the end of the session, a longer second Run meant that there was not always enough time for a longer third Run. However, this problem was later solved when I learned to weave my Penetrating Heaven technique into the Zero Balancing Protocol so that the three Runs are spaced out throughout the session, allowing more time for each Run (see Weaving It Into the Protocol, pages 64-71).

Pause for Thought

In the ZB Protocol, there is not one particular fulcrum that helps to create an expanded state of consciousness for the client. We usually hold each fulcrum for 3-5 seconds and move on, and it is the accumulative effect of many short fulcrums within a session that can result in expanded states.

One day, while I was still developing Penetrating Heaven, I received a Zero Balancing session for myself during which the practitioner happened to do the Toe Sandwich fulcrum on me. This is a fulcrum where you gently 'sandwich' the toes of the client's foot between the fingers of your two flat hands, while your thumbs press your hands together, but not too tightly; you ease off to a comfortable and consistent hold at interface, with attention.

Although not part of the Core ZB Protocol, this is a nice fulcrum hold to do. There is so much available bone in the feet and we hold a lot of our history here. On this occasion the practitioner held the Toe Sandwich for what seemed longer than usual, or longer than I was used to, and I felt myself go into an expanded state of consciousness.

After that I decided to add a long hold Toe Sandwich to my Penetrating Heaven sessions as a precursor or primer, the last thing I did at the feet before going to work at the head. One day a client said that this was what really made her 'drop into it' (her inner journey), what 'set it all off'.

Suddenly I started to have doubts about Penetrating Heaven! Was the effect really due to the Acupuncture point, Tian Chong, GB-9? Or did my clients' journeys simply happen because I was holding the point for a long time - in effect performing a 'skull sandwich' - and introducing a clearer, stronger field into the head and the structures within the skull? (Some brain fulcrums in Secrets of the Skull are longer holding fulcrums with a light touch.)

Could I recreate the same experiences by touching with attention anywhere on the body? For example, could I use the client's foot or a finger to represent their whole body or being? A fulcrum can act locally and globally. That is to say, it can affect the bone at the local site where we are working, and it can have a global effect on the whole body, or the whole person.

Originally, in my own journey, Richard had done what I thought was an HMV at my neck. But later he said that he had put a fulcrum into my Higher Self - so although it seemed like a normal fulcrum, it wasn't. Physically he was still applying the fulcrum at my neck (i.e. locally), but he did it as an offering to my Higher Self (globally), so it had an effect on a different level.

The same applies in Penetrating Heaven. I apply Zero Balancing principles of touch to the point, Tian Chong, GB-9, which lies over the parietal bones of the skull. Although I'm physically touching the client, I'm not working on the parietal bones locally; rather, my focus is on the energy of the points, and I'm working on the level of the mind or the Higher Self of the whole person. Therefore, the effect is more global.

At this point, it seemed that the main keys to help facilitate expanded states of consciousness were: a light touch, with attention; a certain length of time that the fulcrum is held in stillness and constancy, with a slow mindful release; then a certain length of time to allow the effect to play out.

I conceded that any bony part of the body held for a longer time with attention (within a ZB session) may create an expanded state of consciousness because of the characteristic properties of bone (as explained earlier).

However, I remained convinced that using Acupuncture points added another dimension, and had a characteristic influence on the client's experience, due to their particular nature (the "Spirit of the Point").

Moreover, using an Acupuncture point means that I focus my touch and attention on a specific point, whereas the Toe Sandwich covers a larger area that includes several acupuncture points but without making them the focus of the practitioner's attention.

My moments of doubt were part of the development process and they helped me to get clearer on what I was doing. By continuing on my path and offering Penetrating Heaven to many more people, I received plenty of client feedback which proved to me that there is indeed something to Penetrating Heaven, as you will see. I had my method, my technique, it worked, and I was sticking to it!

The Development Process

The development of my Penetrating Heaven technique was often like the dark muddy path of my vision. I didn't always know where it was leading, or how best to proceed. I also didn't know what the Penetrating Heaven experience was like, or how good it was, having not had a session myself, so I relied on client feedback, letting myself be guided by whatever clues appeared.

To get feedback during a session was important but not always easy! I found it difficult to know when to ask the client what was happening, for fear of interrupting their experience. They would often enter a very deep state, from which it is not always easy to speak. Sometimes when I asked them how it was going, all they could manage was a thumbs-up! One client suggested I call them back from their journey by gently sounding a Tibetan bell in order to make the transition back to everyday consciousness gentler and more gradual.

Getting feedback after a session wasn't always easy, either. Clients often told me that their inner experiences were difficult to explain or put into words. ("It's like trying to write about a musical symphony. You can't adequately describe it, you have to experience it.") And they often said that it was unlike anything they had experienced before.

Also, just like after a ZB session, clients would tell me about Penetrating Heaven: "It continues to work for days afterwards." And it can take time to process and digest whatever happened. Many people say that their experience makes more sense a few days later.

Some experiences are deeply personal and private and, for that reason, difficult to share. This was another reason why detailed feedback after a session was not always forthcoming. However, after doing hundreds of sessions on a wide range of people, I have been blessed to receive plenty of feedback, some of which I will include later in this book.

As I offered my technique to more and more people, I found myself being asked more and more challenging questions about my technique and how it works. This forced me to get clearer on what I was doing, and so the field of Penetrating Heaven got clearer, too.

Even though Penetrating Heaven got good responses from the very beginning, and despite growing positive feedback, I lacked confidence that my technique was good enough. That's why I went through a phase of trying to improve it, and get more from it, by adding more to it - adding more complexity to my technique, adding more fulcrums, borrowing brain fulcrums from Secrets of the Skull and any other supporting fulcrums that seemed to enhance the experience, such as the Toe Sandwich.

However, this risked overcomplicating things and - more importantly - overloading the client, because adding too many fulcrums can sometimes leave the client feeling 'wiped out' or depleted. Moreover, dipping in and out of the expanded states can be tiring. Remember: "Less is more!" So I decided to keep these extra fulcrums and techniques in reserve to use if necessary.

Eventually, the sheer weight of feedback convinced me that I really was onto something, so with new confidence I began to relax, and Penetrating Heaven went through a phase of daring to do less.

Thank you, Claire, for insisting "Penetrating Heaven doesn't need improving, it's good enough as it is!"

Now Let's See How Little Zero Balancing We Can Get Away With

Even though my own journey experience had occurred 'outside of' a Zero Balancing session, I wasn't sure if my Penetrating Heaven technique would really work on its own, and so I assumed that it was necessary to do the full ZB Protocol first, in order for the client to become sufficiently relaxed to enter into an altered state of consciousness.

So, in the early days of my research I would begin with a full Zero Balancing session and then simply add Penetrating Heaven onto the end for a total of three consecutive Runs, which was about the limit for an hour-long session, and usually enough for the client.

However, doing the full ZB Protocol meant that there was less time available to explore Penetrating Heaven in more depth, and less time to experiment with longer runs, and it also meant that sometimes the client would become overloaded. Remember, less is more.

I wanted to know the 'minimum effective dose' of Zero Balancing that is necessary in order to achieve the same interesting responses that I had got so far. The answer appeared in the form of a number of new clients who limited the amount of work that I could do on them due to physical challenges that had to be navigated. There was, for example, a reluctance to lie flat on the table, insisting on having a pillow under their back or lying with their knees up, being in chronic pain and hypersensitive to touch, or needing to use the toilet during a session. These challenges all kept my work to a minimum (and tested my attention), but these sessions still got very good responses and feedback, which further boosted my confidence. And I wrote in my journal: "You don't always need much ZB for Penetrating Heaven, probably less than you think."

So, I plucked up the courage to experiment with doing less Zero Balancing - less is more! And I decided to try Penetrating Heaven directly after doing a 10 minute "Evaluatory ZB", which means only doing the evaluations from the ZB Protocol, without any of the fulcrums.

The Evaluatory ZB is still deeply relaxing and can produce the same working signs in the client that occur in a full Zero Balancing session. Such is the power of touch with attention! Doing less Zero Balancing in this way allowed more time to explore Penetrating Heaven.

Sometimes the Evaluatory ZB revealed areas of the skeleton that I felt needed a fulcrum, and so I would go back and add these fulcrums in. But I did only what I felt was necessary.

After doing the Evaluatory ZB I tried my Penetrating Heaven technique, and to my surprise and delight, my clients did indeed go into altered states of consciousness and they also enjoyed journey experiences, although these were not always as deep or as vivid as when I had done the full ZB Protocol.

Using the minimal Evaluatory ZB before Penetrating Heaven gave me more confidence in my technique and proved to me that Penetrating Heaven does indeed work - even with very little ZB.

But, I still wanted to continue doing the full ZB Protocol - and so did my clients! Only now I realized that Penetrating Heaven could be applied a lot earlier in the session. So I stopped using the mini Evaluatory ZB and instead began to learn how to weave Penetrating Heaven into the Zero Balancing Protocol, rather than just adding it onto the end.

Weaving It Into the Protocol - Stage One

Towards the end of the ZB Protocol the practitioner sits at the client's head in order to do some 'passes', i.e. evaluating and then putting in fulcrums in the upper back and neck. And the very last thing we do, right at the end of the Protocol, is the "Closing Sequence" where we work from the head down to the feet in order to finish the session.

Back when I was simply adding my Penetrating Heaven technique onto the end of the Zero Balancing session, I would do so just before the Closing Sequence, partly because it meant that I didn't have to get up from my seat until the end! But also because the client feedback was invariably that not much happened when I did the Closing Sequence before doing Penetrating Heaven. Perhaps this was because the Closing Sequence has an air of completion and feels like the end of the session, as it takes the focus down to the client's feet, with the effect of grounding them. So, I would do Penetrating Heaven just before the Closing Sequence, and that way I had some bodywork left to finish the session, which helped to bring the client back into their physical body.

At that time, I was doing Penetrating Heaven in three consecutive Runs of increasing length, all added onto the end of a ZB session, each Run immediately following the last, one after the other, only pausing for feedback but with no further Zero Balancing in between these Runs.

As I refined my technique, however, I decided it would be better to space the three Runs out, thereby leaving more time in between each Run, and do more Zero Balancing after each Run to help integrate the experience - to actually weave the three Runs strategically into the ZB Protocol with the idea that the experience will go deeper with each Run as the session progresses through the Protocol.

I decided to weave the three Runs into the last part of the Protocol, with the upper back and neck, since I was seated there anyway. So, I would do a Run and then do a pass in the upper back with some fulcrums, or do some work on the neck, before offering another Run.

Sometimes, however, we got so engrossed in Penetrating Heaven - clients usually wanted more - that I was neglecting to do the ZB in the upper back and neck, or I would hesitate to do it for fear of interrupting the client's experience, so I had to make sure I remembered to include it. (In reality, continuing with the ZB Protocol towards the end of a Run did not interfere with the client's experience, especially if I had already done an initial pass in the upper back and the neck evaluations, so that the client's Donkey was used to my hands working there.)

After weaving the three Runs into the last part of the Protocol in this way, I would then do a final pass in the upper back and finish with the Closing Sequence down to the client's feet.

This seemed to work better than merely adding the three Runs onto the end of the ZB Protocol because Penetrating Heaven was now more integrated with the Zero Balancing work.

The next stage in the developmental process was to weave Penetrating Heaven into the Protocol more completely. I had come to think of the three Runs as a beginning, middle and end of the experience, and I was about to discover how to space them out further into the beginning, middle and end of the ZB Protocol, thereby integrating the two approaches even more.

Fully building Penetrating Heaven into a ZB session in this way meant that I didn't do too much work or overload the client, and because I did less work it meant we had more time to do longer Runs, and so the client could get much more from the experience.

Introducing the Dry Run (Later Called the "Intro Run")

By now I had done more and more successful sessions, so I had built up the confidence to offer Penetrating Heaven more widely, although I was conscious of not raising people's expectations too much at the beginning of the session.

Some clients were unsure of exactly when in the session I was doing Penetrating Heaven and when I was doing Zero Balancing, and what the difference was, so I had to learn to explain the sessions better.

One day I offered my friend Mariella a session. While I was waiting for her to arrive at the clinic, I was rehearsing in my mind how to explain Penetrating Heaven to her and decided it would be easier to simply start the session with Penetrating Heaven so that she would know what I was going to do. It would take the mystery out of it, and she wouldn't be lying there waiting in anticipation for me to do this amazing technique sometime in the session. So I omitted the usual seated evaluation. Instead, she lay down straightaway, and I did Penetrating Heaven.

Starting the session in this way also framed it as a Penetrating Heaven session, as distinct to pure Zero Balancing, and helped to set the tone. (Start as you mean to go on!)

But I didn't want to build up too many ideas of what might happen in the session. So in order to manage the client's expectations, and to avoid early disappointment, I decided to play it down and call this a "Dry Run" since we were not really expecting anything to happen. This took the pressure off the client, and off me!

This 'Dry Run' also served as a warm-up or practice run for me, to help me get into the right frame of mind to do Penetrating Heaven, as I was still developing my technique then.

After the Dry Run I would begin the Zero Balancing Protocol with the HMV at the feet (without worrying if it would affect the client's experience like it had in some early trials) and work in the lower back, sacrum and hips, then work down to the feet and repeat the HMV.

Then I came to sit at the client's head to do the HMV at the neck, a pass in the upper back and the neck evaluations, and then do a second Run (thereby weaving it into the Protocol), followed by more Zero Balancing to include all of the upper body work, and then finally do a third Run before finishing with the Closing Sequence.

The Dry Run helped to take the pressure off because it doesn't matter if nothing happens. It's just an introduction, and we will have more Runs to try again later in the session.

So I would tell people that this is just a Dry Run, downplaying it for fear of disappointment, until one day another friend, Trevor, exclaimed: "So that was just a Dry Run, was it?" And he described receiving a rich, colourful, and very meaningful experience already. Wow!

Although people usually need more Zero Balancing to achieve these states, some people have amazing experiences from just the Dry Run, which was a big confidence boost for me.

So now I stopped calling it the "Dry Run" and instead renamed it the "Intro Run". This not only reflected my growing confidence and my belief in the effectiveness of Penetrating Heaven - it also suggests to the client that there will be more Runs to come.

And so I decided to begin each session of Penetrating Heaven by doing the Intro Run first. The Intro Run is the first in a total of three Runs; the other two are woven into a later stage of the ZB Protocol.

The Intro Run

The Intro Run begins a session at the client's head, but this breaks the ZB Protocol, which is a tour of the body in a certain sequence, always mindful of considering the client's Donkey. We start in comparatively less vulnerable areas of the body and only go near the head later on.

I gave a session to my friend Claire, who had had Penetrating Heaven many times before, but this time I started the session with my new Intro Run, without explaining that I had made a change. She wasn't expecting this and it was confusing for her because it was not what she was used to - I had startled her Donkey.

Claire reported that this had been a very different session. More than that, she said that starting off by doing a Run of Penetrating Heaven first had given her a greater awareness and experience of the Zero Balancing than usual. She could feel what the Zero Balancing was doing, and she could feel the energy moving more than she had in previous sessions.

My original 'test pilot' Mike said that the Intro Run allows the person to get a sense of what to expect in a Penetrating Heaven session, both physically and mentally. It gives them a feel for the work, so they know what it is like and what is possible. The client can 'get their bearings' and then decide what they wish to do, so in the next Run they will be prepared and ready. What is more, the Intro Run can give them a taste for the adventure, increasing their enthusiasm for further exploration.

Sometimes the Intro Run is enough for a client to go into an expanded state and have a journey experience. And clients have told me that it continues to work even while I get on with the ZB Protocol. Subsequent Runs then allow the client to go deeper and further with it.

It is as if the Intro Run primes the client; it charges them up and sets the tone for the session, so that the Zero Balancing works for them on *that* level (as well as on the physical). Plus, the Intro Run starts a kind of snowball effect through the session, whereby the Zero Balancing continues to open the client up to the experience of Penetrating Heaven. It is an accumulative process.

Even if a client doesn't go into an altered state this early in the session, the Intro Run can serve as a gauge for me to see how they respond to Penetrating Heaven. It provides early feedback that lets me identify problems or make any adjustments while it is still early in the session. It is also an opportunity for me to give some verbal fulcrums or coaching to assist the client.

In terms of timing, I had previously found that, if something is going to happen in a Run, it will have started within 2 minutes of taking my hands away. Therefore, I decided that in the Intro Run it is only necessary to do just enough to get the ball rolling. I hold the points until I sense a change or notice some working signs - I charge them up and let them go. Then after 2 minutes I simply get on with the ZB Protocol, knowing that Penetrating Heaven is likely to continue working as I do so.

Weaving Penetrating Heaven into the Zero Balancing Protocol like this, i.e. starting the session off with the Intro Run (the first of the three Runs), with the other two Runs following later on, meant that I no longer had to worry so much about how long to give each Run. Although I still took my hands away and waited to allow the client time to have an experience, I was now confident that the Intro Run would continue to work while I carried on with the ZB Protocol. This provided more time and enabled longer second and third Runs.

Weaving It Into the Protocol - Stage Two

To summarise, I decided to begin the session with the Intro Run and then start the ZB Protocol with the HMV (Feet), then work in the lower back, sacrum and hips, and back down to the feet. After that I go back to sit at the head again and do an HMV (Neck), then do a pass in the upper back and the neck evaluations before starting the second Run.

In this way, the client gets used to me working on their neck and back as we approach the second Run. After the second Run I will be going back to do more work on the neck and back, and as the client is used to me working there, it is less likely to startle their Donkey or interrupt the effects of Penetrating Heaven. Also, by doing the neck evaluations before the second Run, I am assessing any neck tension or restriction which, as I later discovered, can be a possible obstacle to the effect of Penetrating Heaven. (See page 156-157)

Sometimes I would check in with the client after the second Run to ask how they were doing, only to find that by talking to them I was interrupting their experience. Talking engages the client's thinking mind and can pull them out of the expanded states of consciousness. I found that it is better to silently continue with the Zero Balancing Protocol first and do a pass in the upper back to bring the client round more gently before I ask how they are doing.

I knew from my own experience of having Zero Balancing that the relaxed dreamlike states can continue quite happily while I receive more bodywork. Fulcrums do not interrupt them but if necessary bodywork can gently bring you back into your body sufficiently for you to be able to talk.

I then continue with another pass in the upper back, and any remaining neck fulcrums, before doing the third Run. In this way I 'fill in the gaps' to complete the Zero Balancing Protocol and fully build Penetrating Heaven into the ZB session.

There was just one more tweak to come which would complete the integration into the Protocol.

The Final Tweak: Alignment

As outlined, I was beginning a session by doing the Intro Run, followed by the ZB Protocol, starting with an HMV (Feet). However, one day I was giving a session to a ZB buddy and, out of habit, and because I was working on a colleague, I started the session with a friendly HMV (Feet) instead. Then in that moment I decided to add a regular HMV (Neck) before doing the Intro Run, and this now became the way I did things. After all, it made sense to align the client on the table first.

I once attended some Acupuncture workshops held by Andrew Nugent-Head. He taught that it is important to always begin Acupuncture by aligning the patient on the table first to ensure better Qi flow. He did this by holding the patient's ankles and pulling with traction, then holding their head and applying traction, then returning to the ankles again.

In fact, when I thought about it, I remembered that for my original journey experience Richard had given me an HMV at my feet first, before the HMV at my neck, but this is so normal in Zero Balancing that it hadn't really registered with me.

So, this was the final tweak in weaving Penetrating Heaven into the Zero Balancing Protocol.

My sessions now look like this: I begin with an HMV (Feet) and an HMV (Neck), followed by the Intro Run (about 2 minutes). After the Intro Run, I continue the ZB Protocol from the lower back, sacrum and hips down to the feet, then do the second HMV (Feet). Next, I sit at the head to do an HMV (Neck), a pass in the upper back and the neck evaluations before doing the second Run (at least 5 minutes). This is followed by another pass in the upper back, and any other fulcrums that I feel are necessary, and then it is time for the third Run (about 10 minutes). Finally, I complete the session with a final pass in the upper back and the Closing Sequence. In this way, I am weaving three Penetrating Heaven Runs into the ZB Protocol.

Relax, Don't Try So Hard, Keep It Simple

Weaving Penetrating Heaven into the Zero Balancing Protocol gave me a better structure to work from. Although later, in the spirit of my own journey along that dark unmarked path, I would venture from the carefully constructed, defined path and work more intuitively.

"Relax" is generally good advice in most situations. I had learned to relax my finger pressure, physically, developing a lighter touch, and as I received more and more positive feedback, my confidence in Penetrating Heaven grew, so I began to relax mentally as well.

I stopped trying so hard. The more we relax, the more we can perceive. And as I began to relax into the process and learned to trust it, so I began to feel more guided by my intuition.

Sometimes during a Run I sensed that the client's experience was beginning to fade. So, without saying anything to them, I touched the points again and repeated the technique, effectively doing several short Runs consecutively to reinforce the effect.

Sometimes I did the Intro Run and then continued with the ZB Protocol in the lower ribs and sacrum, and these fulcrums produced so many working signs that I felt drawn to repeat Penetrating Heaven for an early second Run before resuming the ZB Protocol with the hip and feet fulcrums, and then sit at the head again for the upper body work and the third Run.

Occasionally the second Run can be so productive, with plenty of working signs or positive feedback, that I let it be and allow much more time, and a third Run is not really necessary. Other times it feels right to try a fourth Run. So it is a loose framework, and I adapt and work with the client according to what is happening in the moment. A note from my journal: "Work with the working signs!"

Relaxing and loosening up mentally also helped me to adopt an attitude of experimental play, which led to a freer and more intuitive feel for the work. This led to more discoveries, particularly in terms of how to actually 'do' Penetrating Heaven.

I had already explored the idea of "Less is more" with regard to how much Zero Balancing work was needed for Penetrating Heaven to have an effect, and doing less Zero Balancing gave more time for Penetrating Heaven. Now I wanted to try not only doing less work, but also using less 'technique' in my approach.

Since I was confident that Penetrating Heaven works, I dared to strip away some of the complexity. In other words: "Keep it simple", don't try so hard, and then see if it still works.

To do this, I simplified my technique down to the 'bare bones' of simple touch with attention (Hold, Listen and Allow), while the Stillness Field, silent Om and my Heart Light were kept back in reserve to be used later.

Simple touch with attention became my foundation. From there, I was able to build it up, gradually adding one or more of the various different methods of introducing a clearer, stronger field - the Stillness Field, or silent Om, or Heart Light, and other ideas - later on. Client feedback confirmed it was better to build things up in stages.

Some of these methods of introducing a clearer, stronger field seemed to be more powerful than others, so I came to regard them as like a set of gears for me to use. I could start off simply and step up the process if necessary, going up through the gears as the session progressed.

Some of these gears are based on a few of my other influences, which I will discuss next.

Parallel Breaths

Along with Zero Balancing, Fritz Smith also teaches a simple meditation technique called The Parallel Breath Meditation (which is available on DVD from the Zero Balancing Health Association website). To do this, sit comfortably with your back straight. As you breathe in, feel the breath energy moving from the top of your head down to your base, where you feel your sit bones (Ischium) on the chair. As you breathe out, feel the breath energy moving back up from your base to the top of your head.

In this way the breath energy moves through your body - through the head, the heart and the Hara, through the three Dan Tien (energy centres), or through the body's Chakra System, if you prefer.

These vertical lines of breath energy moving down and up through the body tend to be parallel to each other.

One of the benefits of the Parallel Breath Meditation is that it helps to quieten the 'monkey mind'. As explained earlier, if we do two separate things at the same time and ask the Left Brain to deal with them both, then it is unable to do so and it will go quiet. (In the Parallel Breath Meditation the first of these two things we focus on is the breath pattern, the second thing is how the breath feels as it moves.)

In the second part of the DVD Fritz explains how to use Parallel Breaths on an issue or situation that is bothering you. You place an image of the issue in the energy centre in your lower belly, your lower Dan Tien, and breathe Parallel Breaths through it. You just breathe and feel, and hopefully you will detect a change as things align and get clearer. (For bigger problems, you place the image in front of your Dan Tien, outside of your body.)

When I first learned the Parallel Breath meditation, my understanding was that it was for the practitioner to use for their own benefit, and I do practice it myself. But later I began to wonder if I could use Parallel Breaths during a session for the benefit of the client as well. (See page 160-161)

Running Energy With the Breath

Our breathing affects our energy field, and breathing can be used to focus our attention in the present moment. In therapies such as Medical Qi Gong the practitioner will use their breath, body posture and focused intention to raise their own energy field to a clearer, stronger state in order to help their patient. Similarly some Acupuncturists emphasise the importance of the practitioner's internal state when needling a point.

In Quantum Touch, a healing technique developed by Richard Gordon, the practitioner uses their breath to "run energy" and raise their energetic state to a higher vibration than that of the client, who can then adopt this higher vibration for themselves by a process of 'Entrainment'. This is similar to the effect when a note is played on a piano and a guitar placed near to the piano will sound the same note by simple resonance. The same can be demonstrated using two tuning forks.

Here is an example of 'running energy': Inhale for a count of 4 and imagine energy running up your legs from the Earth and into the rest of your body. Exhale for a count of 4 and imagine the energy flowing from your body - through your arms and hands - to the site of the healing in the client.

Apart from providing a focus for our attention, the breath is also a way to engage our physical body in a very mindful process, thereby uniting the physical with the non-physical.

Clearer, Stronger Fields

Originally I had started with the **Stillness Field** as my clearer, stronger field. Then later it became a **silent Om**, which provided a focus for me as I held the points. In an early trial session, while doing the Stillness Field, I felt my heart opening and filling up with light, which then flowed directly into my hands. This **"Heart Light"** had a power and stillness of its own, so I began to use it. I would touch the points and then visualize my heart open, filled with light, as this light beamed directly into my fingers on the points, as an offering to the client. The responses and feedback were very positive, so this became my favoured method.

I had experimented with doing less Zero Balancing, and now I decided to experiment with less complexity in my Penetrating Heaven technique. Starting with a 'keep it simple' approach, I kept the Stillness Field, the silent Om and my Heart Light back in reserve for me to use in later Runs, if necessary.

And so, for the Intro Run I started simply with touch with attention - Hold, Listen and Allow. This did indeed produce altered state experiences, but not always as deep or as powerful as I was used to, so then in the next Run I would step it up and add the Stillness Field, a silent Om or my Heart Light.

It made sense to start simple, as a gentle introduction to these expanded states, and then build it up gradually in stages with each Run, depending on the client's feedback and responses, using the more powerful methods as we went along - like a set of gears - to take it up a level.

During the pauses I sometimes did Parallel Breaths through me to help me hold the field. One day, while using Hold, Listen, Allow, I found myself doing Parallel Breaths while I was still holding the points, my attention in my fingers, and my client felt that this added something. I was using my breath to help focus my mind and attention, and this seemed to amplify the effect. And so I started to use Parallel Breaths as one of my 'gears' in Penetrating Heaven.

The Parallel Breath Meditation reminds me of the idea in Chinese Philosophy that humans exist "between Heaven and Earth". The vertical lines of breath moving up and down make it easy to imagine that the energy of Earth is being drawn up through the lower body to meet the energy of Heaven as it comes down through the upper body.

One day, while using Parallel Breaths for a Run, I had an experience where I felt or imagined light coming down from Heaven into me, filling my heart, then flowing into my hands, with my fingers on the points. This had a powerful effect on my client, amplifying their Penetrating Heaven experience. So I tried imagining a ball of light above my head flowing down so that I was immersed in a column of light. Then, adapting the idea from Quantum Touch of using the breath to run this energy through me, I tried running energy down from Heaven (instead of the original idea of running energy up from the Earth):

Inhale for a count of 4 as you bring light down from Heaven into you, into your heart; and exhale for a count of 4 as you imagine the light flowing from your heart into your hands. Repeat.

This all became one new technique that I called "Bringing Down the Light from Heaven": I actively imagine light energy coming down from above, into me, with my breath. I actively visualize the light filling me, then combining with my Heart Light and flowing into my hands, with my attention in my fingers on the points. Remembering that it is an offering to the client, I am allowing the light to flow, not forcing it to go anywhere.

I like the idea of light pouring into the gap or 'breathing space' between my fingers and the points (again, as an offering), so that the light can enter the Window of Heaven with all the connotations associated with light: consciousness, enlightening, illuminating, revealing what is hidden. Bringing Down the Light from Heaven seems to be an even more powerful 'gear'. It certainly gets better responses if all else fails to elicit an experience.

So now I had several ways to introduce a clearer, stronger field as I touched the points...

Developing a Set of Gears

Client feedback suggested that the different methods I describe above created different levels of effect: Simple touch with attention (Hold, Listen, Allow) could produce altered state experiences, and using Parallel Breaths seemed to add something to this. Then imagining my Heart Light, or Bringing Down the Light from Heaven, took the experience to a whole new level.

Certainly visualizing light often seemed to make the experience more visual for the client. And their experiences were deeper and more powerful as I stepped it up with each Run, so I came to think of each of these different techniques as like a series of gears to use.

I would begin a session with the Intro Run, for which I would simply use gentle touch with attention (Hold, Listen, Allow) and maybe add Parallel Breaths. Then for the second Run I would perhaps use the Stillness Field, a silent Om or my Heart Light, and finally, for the third Run, Bringing Down the Light from Heaven.

Of course, my choice of method would depend on the client's response. Sometimes, if a particular gear produced a good response, I would use that same gear again for the next Run before stepping it up. A note in my journal: "The Gears are simply options, you don't need to use them all!"

My clients definitely got better responses when I 'changed gear' and built the energy up in this way (with Heart Light and Bringing Down Light from Heaven giving the most powerful responses). In hindsight perhaps this was because the client was already 'warmed up' from having had a previous Run earlier in the session, which made them more receptive to a deeper experience. Also, they have had more of that key ingredient, time. In addition, as each Run is further into the session, the client has also had more Zero Balancing, which all has an accumulative effect.

In the summer of 2013, when I first started developing Penetrating Heaven, I attended a workshop at Gaunts House called "Alchemy of Touch" where Fritz taught that, in order to amplify a fulcrum, you must "get behind yourself more", i.e. you must really engage and focus your attention in your hands. As we know, attention amplifies the effect.

Since each 'gear' is capable of producing an effect, via its own clearer, stronger field, perhaps it is not the particular gear itself that is really so important. It may simply be a means of helping me to quieten my monkey mind and be in the stillness, and focus and hold my attention in my hands in the present moment.

It could also be that my relationship to a particular gear makes it more powerful. Some gears have more personal appeal and they feel more meaningful to me, which adds to the effect. So it is not so much what I'm doing but the fact that I am fully absorbed in it.

When I use my favourite gear, I am fully and wholeheartedly engaged and focused - I "get behind myself" more. Attention amplifies the effect, therefore, the most powerful 'gear' is the one that best keeps my attention in the present moment, so that I 'get out of the way' mentally and allow the process to unfold while holding the field with clear, unwavering focus.

There is more than one way to facilitate these altered state experiences. Earlier I questioned whether they were really induced by the specific Acupuncture point I had chosen. But again, Tian Chong, GB-9, had a personal significance for me.

Other gears work but I felt that Bringing Down the Light from Heaven, via my Heart Light, was the way to go simply because it seemed to give the best experiences for my clients. These became my favourite gears because I associated them with the best feedback.

In practice I generally use my Heart Light for the second Run and then step it up a gear and use Bringing Down the Light from Heaven for the third and final Run. Bringing Down the Light from Heaven incorporates and builds on my Heart Light, because it brings light down from Heaven into my heart (that bit of Heaven in me) and joins with my Heart Light as it flows into my hands and my fingers on the points.

Refining My Technique:
Conscious Touch With Attention

As I continued to develop my technique and my understanding of how Penetrating Heaven works, my appreciation of touch also deepened. There is the physical aspect of touch, such as the degree of pressure (and I had discovered that a light touch is important). And then there is the non-physical aspect of touch, i.e. the significance of attention and consciousness.

Attention amplifies the effect of our touch. As they say in the practice of Qi Gong: "Qi flows where our attention goes", and I would add... "provided that our touch is light enough to *allow* the Qi to flow."

I had established that the two main aspects for achieving the best effect are a lighter touch (touch with attention - consciousness is key!) and timing (holding for a longer time, in stillness, in the present moment, followed by a slow, mindful release; then waiting and allowing a long enough pause for the effect to unfold).

One of my case studies to certify in Zero Balancing was a woman who was surprisingly sensitive and seemed to flinch in pain at the slightest pressure. This made me ease off my finger pressure and pay more attention, adopting what I called "Bomb Squad" mode, i.e. working slowly and carefully just in case she 'went off' without warning. As an eager student I was disappointed because I thought I was hardly doing anything and barely touching her. But she loved it and showed lots of working signs. This was an early lesson for me that attention is a key.

'Safecracker' is probably a better description than 'bomb squad' - that level of careful listening and attention. Really, this is about working carefully with the client's Donkey. There may be a history of trauma or abuse - you never know what you are dealing with. Therefore, it is better to begin with a light touch, and you may be able to go deeper later in the session, or in a future session.

The power of touch lies not just in the physical aspect of touch. It includes one's mind and attention as well. I am touching the client with my mind through my fingers and not merely physically. As my pressure eases off, it is as if I am touching the person more with my attention than with my fingers. The key is keeping one's mind (one's conscious awareness) in one's fingertips the whole time.

I had several clients suffering with poor sleep and I started applying these same principles to an Acupuncture point called An Mian ("Peaceful Sleep"), which is located behind each ear. One of these clients was a 2-year-old boy. His mum held him facing me while I stood in front of him and reached behind his head to locate the points. As I touched the points, he stared at me intently the whole time, and nothing seemed to be happening. I was slightly distracted by his innocent gaze but as soon as I refocussed my attention and put all of my mind in my fingertips - Bingo! He was out like a light, and asleep in his mother's arms. This again highlights the importance of one's conscious attention in touch.

As I said earlier, Acupuncture points provide us with certain possibilities but their effect depends on how we engage the point - the technique, the quality of touch, the timing, and there is also the effect of the mind. Consciousness is key! The attention of the practitioner, and perhaps also that of the client, has an effect.

A 2017 study from the Department of Neuroscience at the University in Chieti, Italy, found that there are differences in brain activity between clients who receive mindful touch and those who receive non-mindful touch, i.e. when the therapist is focused on something else.

One time, while having a massage, I noticed that the therapist's hands felt hotter when she did some moves compared to others. She explained that this was when she was using more focused intention. Again, this shows there is more to touch than merely performing a physical move.

Refining My Technique: Finding the Right Level of Touch

I knew that my Penetrating Heaven technique required a lighter touch with more attention and I reasoned that the right level of touch must lie somewhere between the bone and thin air (or the aura). Like in the story of Goldilocks and the Three Bears, there are three levels of touch: too heavy, too light and just right. So, I am really trying to find the sweet spot in between.

I found that the best way to find the right level of touch is to start with definite physical contact on the point, nestling in gently to get a good bone-to-bone connection. I do this just briefly, enough for the client to know that I'm there, as if I am 'knocking at the door' to say hello. Then I immediately but gradually start to ease off to a lighter, more optimal level of touch.

So, starting from bone as my base, I begin to ease off into a lighter touch, gradually reducing my finger pressure while increasing my attention in order to maintain the connection with the points. In this way, little by little, I find a level of light touch that is comfortable and optimal for achieving the desired effect. Having found this sweet spot, I apply my technique and hold for a sufficient length of time.

This lighter touch allows more to happen because it creates a gap or 'breathing space' that enables the technique to work, and allows the client to respond. Like the analogy of the boat moored in the harbour, this 'wriggle room' gives the energy the freedom to move.

To be clear, I am not taking my finger off the point entirely. I create a thin 'gap' between my finger and the point, but there is still a connection. I imagine it as like a spark gap for an electrical spark to jump between two electrodes or contacts. And in this space, the thin gap between the point and my finger, is where the magic happens.

I have done Penetrating Heaven through thick hair, and even a wooly hat (it still works!) Perhaps this helped by acting as a buffer that created the space for something to happen. Earlier I told the story of doing Acupressure on Pamela, using Yun Men, LU-2, Cloud Gate. Because of her condition, I didn't use very firm pressure and settled into a gentle touch as I held the points. And again, her layers of clothing may have served as a buffer that helped to keep my fingers sufficiently off the points to create the level of touch that was required for her to have the experience of flying through clouds.

In Acupressure, we usually apply firm finger pressure deep into the skin. This physical action is generally used for physical complaints, i.e. this heavier level of touch works more on a physical level. In my understanding, the finger pressure 'depresses' the energy of the point, then upon release of the finger the energy 'springs back' and comes up again to reassert itself. (This may partly explain the phenomenon I observed in the early trials, where clients fed back that nothing happened until I took my hands away: 'Charge me up and let me go!') Acupressure is forceful and imposes something on the physical body. It works on the basis that an action results in a reaction.

In contrast, Penetrating Heaven is less physical. It uses a lighter touch with more attention, and works more on the level of the mind. Instead of performing an action, I simply meet the point as it is, in stillness. I am not imposing anything, I am offering to connect, like saying hello. Therefore, the point doesn't react (since it has nothing to react against) but rather responds and expresses on its own terms. I listen to it rather than telling it what to do. It is a different relationship, with a different effect.

If you jump into a lake, then you make waves and disturb the stillness of that environment; however, if you gently ease yourself into the water, then the lake can receive you and reveal itself, as it is.

As I said earlier, the Chinese names for the Acupuncture points can refer to several things simultaneously. The points can access different aspects of us, both physical and non-physical, depending on how we engage with them. Therefore, different levels and qualities of touch can produce different effects.

Refining My Technique: The Sweet Spot in the Spark Gap

So, to do Penetrating Heaven, I locate the points, touch bone base, and then I start to ease off my finger pressure immediately - but slowly and gradually, with focused attention - in order to allow a thin gap under my fingers, where I find the sweet spot, the optimal level of touch. (Note: The optimal level of touch is not fixed. It is alive and it can vary and change over time. Also, this sweet spot is different for different people, and it can change for the same individual from one session to another.)

As I ease off into a lighter touch, with my mind and attention in my fingertips, it is a case of how light I can go while still maintaining my connection to the points, i.e. without losing the connection.

Imagine you are dipping your finger into a bowl of syrup and slowly lifting it out. Your finger is still joined to the syrup in the bowl by a golden thread that clings to your finger as you lift off. Likewise, as I start to ease off the pressure and lift my finger off the point, I try not to lose the connection or break the 'thread' with the points, until I decide it is time to release and take my hands away.

If I do lose the connection, I can always start again. And the Intro Run at the beginning of the session can be used to explore the optimal level of touch for each individual client.

By using a lighter touch I am using more attention, and through this attention I can sense when I have found the optimal level of touch. With practice and experience I could perceive the sweet spot that lies in the 'spark gap', the place where the magic happens.

It is like driving a car. As you ease off the clutch pedal while pressing the accelerator, there is a 'bite' that occurs as the gear engages, and a change in the engine sound tells you that you are in business. Similarly, with Penetrating Heaven, I touch the points and ease off my finger pressure, thereby opening up the spark gap that is necessary for something to happen. As I hit the sweet spot, the right level of touch, I usually notice a subtle 'bite', or a subtle change in feeling. (As I say, this was a later development, an intuitive sense that came with practice and experience.)

When I feel the 'bite', I know I am at the sweet spot in the gap, i.e. I am at the right level of touch for the effect to kick in. This is where I pause and hold the points.

Sometimes the bite may be accompanied by working signs, for example rapid eye movements or changes in the client's breathing and/or facial expression. So I watch for working signs as I ease off.

This is where I introduce a clearer, stronger field to the points by using one of my gears.

I hold the points at this level of touch and apply my technique, with my chosen gear, for a sufficient length of time until I am sure that something is happening for the client. Again, sensing this is intuitive but it gets easier with practice and experience, and by watching the working signs. With my mind in my fingertips I may sometimes ask myself mentally: "What is happening? Should I come off, should I stay on?" And I will get a sense of what to do.

Once I am sure that the process is well underway, I can start to slowly release the points.

Refining My Technique: A Slow, Mindful Release

It is not only the quality of touch that is important. The way you release the points is, too. As I developed a lighter touch with more attention, I also adopted a slow, gradual, mindful Release, as if I take my fingers away stealthily so that I don't disturb what is happening.

In the early trials clients had told me: "Nothing happens until you take your hands away" because when my touch was too heavy it acted as a brake. This led to me developing a lighter touch, and with a lighter touch things began to happen while I was still holding the points. But then, for some clients, when I took my hands away the inner experience would cease. ("It stopped when you took your hands away!") At first I assumed that my touch was now too light, so that perhaps there was not enough meaningful connection to reliably send the client on their journey. It was more likely, however, that I had released the points either too quickly or too soon, i.e. before the effect had had time to be fully established. Therefore, I needed to stay on the points and 'charge them up' for longer.

This illustrated to me that the right *timing* of holding and release is key. Knowing when and how to release is just as important as the *quality* of touch and attention. You cannot stay on the points for too long, especially with a heavy touch, because this blocks the effect. At the same time, you cannot release the points too quickly or leave the sweet spot too soon, i.e. before the client's inner experience sets in. Generally, I start the Release when I'm confident that something is happening and that my client's journey is well underway.

For a while it seemed that, if my client had had several sessions of Penetrating Heaven before, or if they were particularly sensitive and accustomed to meditation and journeying, they didn't need me to hold the points for quite as long, so I would start the slow, gradual Release immediately. But later I found that clients could show the opposite response in another session, so I concluded that the response depends on the person and where they are at on the day.

It seems that, rather than being fixed, the client's sweet spot can move and vary between sessions. If it is closer to the bone, a heavier touch may still work, whereas if it is further out from the skin, a lighter touch is required to find that sweet spot and engage with it.

I had also considered whether the client's response - in other words, the distance at which the sweet spot is found - may depend on the condition of the points, i.e. whether the points feel open or closed. But I have not researched this further because in practice you can simply use the Intro Run to determine the client's response to your level of touch. You can also do two Intro Runs, one with a more physical touch and one with a less physical touch. Depending on which one is more responsive, that is the level of touch you should aim for in the later Runs.

If the client shows working signs while my fingers are still on the points, I may hold there for a little longer to make sure things are well underway before I begin the Release.

If the effect stops when I take my hands away, the client may show signs of 'snapping out of it' such as taking a breath, gently shaking their head, or repositioning their body on the table. So, work with the working signs. If you are not sure what is happening, ask the client for feedback and repeat the Run.

If things are going well, the working signs will often increase after I take my hands away. Then I will simply sit back and wait, allowing the client to enjoy their experience of the Run.

By starting off quite 'physically' and then easing off into a lighter touch, it is as if I leave an 'energy imprint'. And because the Release is almost imperceptibly slow and gentle, the client often won't notice that I have taken my hands away. Clients often tell me that they can still feel my fingers on the points even when I have fully released. This is a sensation that some people like, perhaps because it feels reassuring. It gives a sense of contact or connection. It might also provide a focus for the client that enables them to put *their* attention into the points if they choose, although this is not something I instruct them to do.

The Awareness Zone

(How Far Out Does It Get?)

When I trained in the Emmett Technique, Ross Emmett spoke of "The Awareness Zone", the area just off the physical body that is still our space, and where we still have a certain degree of awareness. He explained that, because of this Awareness Zone, a horse knows to kick you even though you are outside of its field of vision!

Some of the practitioners on my course used the Emmett Technique to work on horses, and I was struck by their lightness of touch. They told me that a horse will respond if they do the Emmett Technique in thin air, i.e. just off the horse's body, without physically touching the animal.

When practising the Bowen Technique, with my client lying face down, if I place my hands on their back too quickly, sensitive clients may flinch when I touch their skin. However, if I pause and let my hands hover just above the skin for a moment before moving gradually closer with careful attention, the client will remain relaxed when I touch them physically. The point is that we don't end at skin level. Our energy field extends out from the body.

If we go on the premise that every body has this "Awareness Zone", many things start to make sense. The Awareness Zone helps us to visualize and understand what is happening.

Picture the Awareness Zone as it extends a short distance from the skin. Now imagine that there are different spatial layers extending out from the body into the Awareness Zone, that respond to different levels of touch. The sweet spot lies somewhere in there. The exact location can vary - sometimes the sweet spot is closer to the bone whereas at other times it can be further out. Occasionally it is actually so far out that I am not physically touching the skin at all; my fingers are merely hovering in the client's hair space just off the points.

This helps to explain the variety of responses. Sometimes a client's experience starts to happen immediately when I start touching the points, while at other times it takes a bit more time for the effect to kick in because I am still easing off into the sweet spot; and sometimes nothing happens until I take my hands away.

The idea of the Awareness Zone also helps to explain the client's sensitivity around the quality and timing of touch. As you already know, if my touch is too heavy, or if I take my fingers away too slowly, the client's inner journey can be inhibited. Likewise, if I take my fingers away too early, before the effect is fully established, then this can 'break the spell'. And if I take my fingers away too abruptly, it creates a disturbance in the Awareness Zone, which can disrupt or end the client's experience. (This is why a slow, mindful Release is important.)

Practitioners of different disciplines have suggested to me that the different levels of our being - our physical body, our mental body and our emotional body - can be accessed through different spatial levels of touch, and that the more subtle aspects of us can be accessed through a more subtle quality of touch.

Perhaps working at different levels of touch within the Awareness Zone not only determines the nature of the effect but also where the effect takes place. One practitioner said that when you physically touch someone, the body assumes that you are working on that particular local area, i.e. the place where you touch, whereas if you hold your hands just off the body and hover over the skin, the effect will be more global.

On this subject, a Reflexologist once told me that during her training she learned about "Linking", where the practitioner doesn't touch the client's foot but holds one finger over the top of the foot and one finger off the sole of the foot so that the fingers point at each other. The idea is that the two fingers 'connect' in the space in between and affect the field there, in this case the client's foot. I have tried this idea on clients who had painful areas that they did not want me to touch and some clients have found relief even though I did not touch them.

Part Two

In Part One I described my journey of discovery and the development of my technique of Penetrating Heaven. In Part Two I will explore how to apply my technique for the purpose of self-development and healing, using case examples and client feedback with accounts of some of my client's inner journey experiences to illustrate what is possible...

The Quest for Answers

Initially when I started working with Penetrating Heaven, the idea was simply to "see what happens". And indeed plenty did happen. Most people had some sort of experience, and these were often visual and usually interesting.

However, as I satisfied myself that Penetrating Heaven 'works', i.e. that it has an effect in its own right in addition to the effects of Zero Balancing, and as I gained more confidence in my technique, I began to wonder: What else is possible? What can we use this for?

I felt sure that there was more to these altered states of consciousness than just random waking dreams, and I wanted to see whether the experiences that Penetrating Heaven elicited could be relevant, meaningful and of practical use to people. Perhaps they offered access to helpful insights and information.

We know that in Zero Balancing clients may enter altered states of consciousness from which ideas, inspiration and new perspectives can bubble up during a session.

In my journey with Richard Walters, the 'Frame' had simply been to "see what happens" but the inner experience that unfolded seemed to relate to my life situation at the time and a particular question that I was mulling over in the back of my mind. Having just certified in Zero Balancing, I felt at a crossroads in my career and wondered: "What next?" And then in my journey I saw the two paths. So the question was in my mind and the answer appeared (and I interpreted my experience through the lens of what was going on in my life at the time).

I now decided to experiment with using a Frame. I would have the client set an intention that their Penetrating Heaven experience would relate to a particular area of their life, for example their career or their relationship. This quickly led to clients putting specific questions into their Frame. (The client would then let their question go and 'see what happens'.)

I wanted to know if framing the session in this way could provide a focus for the altered states of consciousness, and whether any 'bubble-ups' that occurred would relate to the client's question.

Putting a question into the Frame focuses the client's intention as we begin the session, and it gives them a specific reference point from which to interpret their experience at the end of the session.

Zero Balancing can put us in touch with stillness. And just as stillness helps to settle a glass of muddy water and bring clarity, so it can help to settle a mind clouded by thoughts.

My idea was for the deep relaxation offered by Zero Balancing to quieten the conscious, thinking mind (the 'monkey mind' or ego mind), so that the client can get out of their own way mentally. Then Penetrating Heaven (Tian Chong) opens the client to the influence of Heaven (Tian), bringing more clarity and insight. You create the right conditions... and then answers appear.

I see Penetrating Heaven as me introducing a clearer, stronger field specifically at the point Tian Chong and creating a Still Point around which the energy of the point can re-organize itself. One could imagine this as the client's thoughts about their framed question having an opportunity to re-organize, thereby creating space for new thoughts and new perspectives to arise.

Our inner knowing is sometimes referred to in the saying: "I feel it in my bones." What better way could there be to access this inner knowing than by using Zero Balancing. As the art of touching bone, it is the perfect springboard to experiencing what is inside of us!

The Answers Are Within You

Many scientists have made famous discoveries or had ground-breaking realisations while they relaxed. Kekulé fell asleep by the fire and dreamed of the chemical structure of the benzene ring. Archimedes famously had his "Eureka!" moment in the bath and was not the last great mind to claim that inspiration came to him in the hot tub.

Most of us will have had the experience of having a question and searching for an answer (or trying to remember something we have forgotten). We think hard and strive and, failing to come up with the answer, we give up on our quest. We let it go and go out for a walk or do the washing up, and then suddenly the answer appears to us from the depths of our sub-conscious mind.

The same thing happened to me when I was searching for Acupuncture points to help facilitate inner journey experiences. As I described earlier, the question of which point to use was in my mind that day in the park. But I let it go, lay down in the sun, and relaxed - only for the idea to 'pop into my head', or bubble up from within, to use Tian Chong, GB-9, Penetrating Heaven.

So I started to work with a simple premise:

The answers to your questions are within you...
(And the answers come to you in stillness.)

This idea is supported by sages and teachers:

"There is nothing outside of us. It's all in us."
- Yogi Bhajan

"The Universe is not outside of you. Look inside yourself; everything that you want, you already are."
- Rumi

"Your mind will answer most questions if you learn to relax and wait for the answer."
- William S. Burroughs

"Quiet the mind and the soul will speak"
- Ma Jaya Sati Bhagavati

The answers we seek can come to us when we relax, let go, and 'get out of our own way'. Zero Balancing is a great way to relax the body and the mind, and from this space 'bubble-ups' occur.

In his book "Stillness Speaks", Eckhart Tolle says that stillness is our "essential nature" and he talks of the "profound wisdom that is to be found in stillness". "*Wisdom comes from the ability to be still... Being still... activates the non-conceptual intelligence within you.*"

Tolle also says: *"Stillness is where creativity and solutions to problems are found."* This suggests to me that the stillness of a ZB fulcrum - or of one of my 'gears' in Penetrating Heaven - can give rise to insights, inspiration and answers.

So far I have discussed *stillness*, which is first and foremost an inner quality. By contrast, *silence* is an outer condition. Although not essential, silence can be helpful in tapping into our inner wisdom, too. As someone once said: "Silence isn't empty, it's full of answers." Most of a Zero Balancing session will be done in silence.

Albert Einstein knew the value of silence, and the power of the pause:

*"I think ninety-nine times and find nothing.
I stop thinking, swim in silence, and the truth comes to me."*
- Albert Einstein

Another interesting quote from Albert Einstein:

"We can't solve problems by using the same kind of thinking we used when we created them."

As I mentioned earlier, in Zero Balancing the expanded states of consciousness can lead to the client being less well held in their dysfunctional patterns, which may cause them to shift out of their current thinking. As a result, many clients experience a new perspective and see things in a different way.

Framing the Session (Explaining Penetrating Heaven: What It Is and How It Works)

Each session should begin by making a good Donkey Connection with the client in order to build trust. It is helpful to spend a few minutes explaining to the client what to expect. (This is done while still face to face with the person, before they lie down on the massage table.)

I start by talking about Zero Balancing, what it involves, that it is deeply relaxing and that it can help us to access altered states of consciousness, like a relaxed meditative state. Then I introduce Penetrating Heaven and the simple premises it is based on, which are:

1. The answer to your question is within you.

2. This answer can come to you and bubble up from your sub-conscious mind if you are able to relax in body and mind, 'get out of your own way' mentally, and let go.

3. Zero Balancing is a great way to relax both your body and mind, and it can offer you the opportunity to open up to new possibilities: physically, mentally and emotionally. And then Penetrating Heaven takes this a step further.

I go on to explain: "Penetrating Heaven is a technique where I touch points on the sides of your head while you are in a relaxed state in order to give you focus and clarity, so that your answers can come."

I was pleasantly surprised by how many clients readily and instinctively agree with the idea that the answers are within us. There is a shared sense that there is something beyond our normal waking consciousness - whether we see that something as our sub-conscious mind, our Higher Self, or the 'wisdom within' - and that it is possible for us to access it.

Then I explain the idea of the Frame, which gives a structure or a 'container' for the session. It is an opportunity for the client to set their intention for the session. This can be in the form of a question or a problem, or a situation in their life that they would like more clarity on. (The Frame still also includes a discussion about any physical issues the client may have.)

The Frame helps to focus the session and sets a direction for the client. It could be argued that it plants a seed - a suggestion and an expectation of an answer - as I invite the client to put a question in the Frame before they lie down on the massage table. I will discuss verbal fulcrums and the power of suggestion later. (See page 99-100)

Sometimes the invitation to put a question in the Frame can make the client feel as though they have been 'put on the spot' and they feel under pressure to think of a question. For this reason I explain: "If you don't have a question, that's okay. You can simply 'dive in and see what happens', and perhaps one will occur to you as you are lying there. If it does, ask it silently to yourself."

"But if you do have a question about any area of your life - career, relationships, health - then now is the opportunity to place it in the Frame and set your intention for the session. Then let your question go and know that the answer may bubble up during the session."

Zero Balancing helps create expanded states of consciousness while Penetrating Heaven provides a focus; it couples the expanded state with a particular direction in the form of the client's question, i.e. their intention for the session. This gives the client a context to relate their inner experience to, helping them to interpret what occurs for them.

Interestingly, I found that the client's question needs to be phrased in a particular way, which I will discuss next.

How to Frame the Question

A wise man once said:

"The quality of your life depends on
the quality of the questions you ask yourself."

It is important how you word your question. At the end of one of my early sessions a client told me: "I think I asked the wrong question!" Some coaching may be required before the work begins.

The first thing is to ask an open question, i.e. not a question with a Yes/No answer, because the situation is often not that simple, even if the client thinks it is. The answer could instead be: "It depends!"

The second thing is, it needs to be made clear that Penetrating Heaven is not fortune-telling. Therefore it is best for the client not to ask what will happen in the future but rather to ask about their present situation.

While the question provides a focus for the session, it should still be an open question or a line of enquiry about a particular situation, not too limited or too defined.

Experience has taught me that the best question seems to be: "What do I need to know [about my specific situation]?"

Some clients have come up with their own variations of this, such as:
"What do I need to focus on?"
"What is happening with…?"

Quite often clients feel stuck in a particular situation and their question may be: "What is stopping me from…?" If they get an answer early in the session, they can then ask: "What can I do about it?" Often people want to know "What should I do?" But sometimes the answer is not to do anything and instead to wait, or to let go, so I suggest rephrasing it to: "What is my next step?"

Some clients may prefer a theme rather than a direct question. One client told me that she preferred to use "I wonder..." as a more open invitation for insights to bubble up around her chosen subject.

Sometimes a client may be brave enough to ask one of the Fundamental Questions of Life, such as "Who am I?" or "Why am I here?", seeking direction with "What is my purpose?" or "What should I do with my life?", or seeking purpose and inspiration with "What would I love to create?" or "What wants to come into being through me?"

Initially I invited my clients to frame their question either by stating it to me out loud or by writing it down, because I thought that articulating the question would help them to set their intention. But this is not necessary. The client's question (and the answer) is private. They do not need to share it with me, and very few people do.

Sometimes the client does not have a specific question and they just prefer to dive in and "See what happens", with a spirit of adventure and the attitude of an explorer. Of course, even without a Frame or a Question, Penetrating Heaven still has an effect, only the client does not have that specific reference or 'hook' to hang their experience on afterwards. Nevertheless, they generally find that their journey is still meaningful and relevant to their current life situation, and it often relates to something that was on their mind anyway.

I once had a client who was well aware of her situation but she was all out of questions, so she simply asked for help from that still space which Penetrating Heaven takes you to.

Some clients ask for a pen and paper at the end of their session because they feel the need to write down - or draw - the answers, insights and ideas that bubbled up for them. This helps to capture the journey because, as with dreams, if you don't write your experience down or solidify the memory in some way, it may be lost as you return to everyday consciousness. For this purpose, I started to offer a 'capture sheet' and I mention this to the client at the start of the session.

Verbal Fulcrums and the Power of Suggestion

Zero Balancing involves very little talking. Apart from discussing the Frame at the beginning, few words are spoken during a session. However, it is important for the practitioner to be mindful of what they *do* say because, while receiving Zero Balancing, the client can go into an expanded state of consciousness and therefore become more suggestible. For this reason, one should only use positive phrases, or carefully chosen Verbal Fulcrums.

Hypnotherapy and Neuro-Linguistic Programming (NLP) are not my area of expertise but a few of my clients have suggested these therapies could be combined with Zero Balancing to leverage off the altered states of consciousness and suggestibility. Other clients have told me that they use ZB sessions to silently repeat mantras or affirmations, consciously availing themselves of their more open and expanded state.

At first, I did not like to say too much about Penetrating Heaven at the start of the session because I did not want to influence the client's experience. Moreover, I wanted to prove that Penetrating Heaven works in its own right, i.e. that the effects cannot just be put down to the power of suggestion.

However, in order to get the best out of a session it may be necessary to explain a few things during the framing stage, otherwise clients may get confused about what is 'supposed' to happen and when. And sometimes it may require a bit of coaching to guide the client in their session.

One of the problems with inviting questions is that it can create pressure to get an answer! Especially in the early days, when I was unsure whether Penetrating Heaven would really work, I did not want to build up expectations too much in case the client was disappointed. On the other hand, inviting questions creates a positive suggestion that answers will come, especially with the promise of a capture sheet at the end of the session which suggests that something is going to happen and there will be something for the client to write down afterwards.

In the end, I could not totally avoid using suggestion, so I decided to embrace it and use positive language to build a good Donkey Connection and help the client to be open.

Although I did not write a 'script' for leading my clients through Penetrating Heaven, I did find myself tending to repeat the same phrases each time. These evolved from my client's feedback and from answering their questions.

Repeating the same ritual and routine each time is important, even if (actually, especially if) the client has had a session before because it builds an association with the experience, which sets things up to be reinforced when I come to use the same phrases again in future.

The ZB Protocol soon becomes familiar to the client and helps their Donkey to feel safe because they know the kind of thing that's going to happen. And because they know what to expect, they can relax and get into the session more quickly. This is true of Penetrating Heaven as well.

Tips for Framing the Session

Framing the session helps the client to feel safe, to know what to expect, to orientate themselves and to make the most of the experience. Over time I learned how to Frame the session in order to avoid some common obstacles. Here are a few things to remember:

Future Pacing the client's Donkey

Having explained the idea behind Penetrating Heaven - i.e. that the answers are within and, if we relax and get out of the way, they can bubble up and arise into our awareness - I then talk about the procedure and what is going to happen. This is important for new clients but I learned to do this for returning clients, too. Even if someone has had a session before, they may not remember how it goes, which is why it is important to treat it like their first session, framing and explaining the procedure to reinforce it again. This will future pace their Donkey, so they know what to expect. This is also a good opportunity to address potential problems and common obstacles, some of which I will talk about here.

Permission to speak, Sir

Because I don't speak while doing Zero Balancing, I found that some clients worry about interrupting me as I work. Therefore it can be good to explain to the client beforehand that I won't speak much during the session but that they are free to speak at any time if they are unsure about anything or if they feel uncomfortable in any way.

Some clients are concerned that, if they speak during the session, they will 'break the spell' or interrupt the process, so I reassure them that I can always repeat the technique and take them back to where they left off. (This also applies if I happen to interrupt their altered state experience when I check in with them.)

No limits!

In the beginning I assumed that clients would limit themselves to asking only one question. However, I then found that some clients would go into a session with more than one question, sometimes relating to more than one issue. Sometimes you may receive an answer early in the session and I encourage more questions to explore the issue further or to address another issue. You are allowed to ask more questions while lying there!

I found myself using permissive language such as "Just allow yourself to...", or "You may choose to...". The word "allow" suggests that you have permission for something to happen; it makes it okay for it to happen. "You may" is a phrase that offers permission and implies choice; it can open up possibilities. "Choose to" is a phrase that encourages or guides the client in a direction without applying force or pressure.

Plenty of opportunities

I discovered that some people think they only have one chance to get the answer, so I reassure my clients that we have several Runs at it: "Don't worry if you don't get anything at first. You will have more than one go at it. We will start with an Intro Run (and you may or may not get anything from that). The idea is that the Zero Balancing bodywork relaxes you and takes you deeper over the course of the session, and you will have several goes at receiving something. Each time you go deeper, so you will probably receive more as the session goes on. There is plenty of time for several attempts."

Don't try so hard - Just let it happen

Some clients try too hard, repeating their question to themselves as they lie there, almost like a mantra. For example, James, one of my clients, realised that he kept asking his question "on a loop" but that this was actually blocking the answer. Because of this, I advise my clients to ask their question and then let it go. It is not necessary to keep repeating your question. Simply ask it at the beginning (or write it down), in order to set your intention, and then just let the question go. It's like ordering something online: You click on your item and expect that it will come. You don't keep ordering it! Be patient and trust your sub-conscious mind to deliver. Let go of the question and allow yourself to receive the answer. I reassure my clients that they don't have to do anything. They can just relax and let me do the work.

Capturing the experience while it's fresh

Finally, I tell the client that at the end of the session there will be a capture sheet for them to scribble down bullet points, doodles or ideas because otherwise their inner journey can easily slip away. It's just like when you have a dream: You wake up, go to the bathroom, and the dream is forgotten, unless you capture it right away.

Be Open to Receiving Answers

In Zero Balancing we talk of the 'blank sheet', i.e. having an open mind, without expectations. I want my client to be open to receiving the experience of Penetrating Heaven and to embrace the mystery.

A client of mine, an actress, once noted: "Get out of your own way, that's what we say in show business!" There is also the saying: "You've got to lose yourself to find yourself." Essentially, you give up control to a process bigger than you.

In the early days I would tell people "Just go with whatever happens", until one client said that this made it sound like a 'ghost train' scenario! It is therefore important to choose your words carefully so that the client feels safe enough to be open.

The dream journey worker Robert Moss asks in one of his guided meditations: "Are you ready for an adventure, yes?" That is a positive suggestive question, as is: "Are you open to that?" Such phrasings are helpful because they encourage a spirit of adventure, an attitude that lets the client "dive in and explore". And that is essentially what we want.

The client needs to be open to receive whatever may happen and be willing to engage with it, and accept their answer in whatever form it comes. So expect nothing, welcome everything!

I heard a story of a man who was meditating in order to meet his spirit guide but during his meditation he saw a vision of an exotic dancer. He tried to ignore it but the image persisted until finally he asked: "Who are you? What do you want?" She replied: "I'm your spirit guide, I'm trying to get your attention!"

In one of my sessions, I leant closer to my client on the table and asked her quietly in a soft voice: "How are you doing? Do you feel that you are starting to get any answers yet?" And the lady replied: "Oh I f*cking know the answer! I'm just avoiding it!"

We cannot assume that we know what is going to happen or how our answer will unfold. We must drop expectations that things will be a certain way, and we must not compare our experience to previous sessions or other types of journey we may have had. Instead, we must but be willing to enter into something new.

So perhaps the best phrase to encourage openness in the client is the one from my original experience with Richard: "See what happens." And I might also add: "If you think nothing is happening yet, don't worry." This frames it up in a way that makes it okay for 'nothing to happen', while at the same time I explain that something can happen later on. It is possible for people to start getting answers straight away, yet it may need a little more time, or a little more bodywork, to help the client to relax into an altered state of consciousness.

Sometimes you get the full answer straight away, and it can be a dramatic revelation. At other times you only get a clue, or the next piece of the puzzle, or the next step to take.

Sometimes the answer may occur to you later that day, or in a few days - some clients say that a session continues to unfold for several days. Simply take what comes and see if it makes sense later.

The answers are within you, but not necessarily in the form you might expect. I explain that the language of the sub-conscious mind is often symbolic or metaphorical. Answers may come in many forms: as images, symbols, thoughts, words, sounds, songs, memories, movie scenes, emotions or physical sensations. There is no right or wrong way to experience this; it is not supposed to be a particular way. So let go of any attachment to the outcome. Be open to receiving and see what happens.

(Note: When answers come in the form of physical sensations, it can be useful to ask: "What is your body trying to tell you?" Do these sensations remind you of any physical complaints you may have felt in the past?")

Diving Into the Intro Run

Before the client lies down on my massage table, I have explained what Zero Balancing is and what Penetrating Heaven is, and framed a question, so now it's time for the Intro Run.

The Intro Run helps to build a good Donkey Connection because it is a gentle introduction to Penetrating Heaven. It offers a preview of what the process will be like, thereby helping to ease any apprehension about entering the unknown before the session gets fully underway.

The Intro Run can help to identify any potential obstacles to the experience early on in the session. It can also help to remove the pressure on the client to have an experience. (The client knows that there will be more Runs, and more opportunities to have an experience, later in the session.)

If it is appropriate, I may offer the client a blanket, as some people like to have a feeling of being cocooned in comfort and safety before entering into an altered state of consciousness.

I begin with an HMV at the feet, then sit behind the client's head and do an HMV at the neck. This is a good opportunity to explain a few things to the client while they are still 'with me', so that I won't have to talk too much later on when they are in an expanded state.

I explain that I'm about to touch the Penetrating Heaven points at the sides of their head, and that it's just an introduction for them to know how it feels and what to expect later on.

I explain that some people start to get answers straightaway but that they shouldn't worry if they don't get anything yet, reminding them that we have plenty of time for more attempts throughout the session. I mention that, as I do more Zero Balancing, they will go deeper, and so they will receive more answers as the session goes on.

As I offered more sessions of Penetrating Heaven, I found myself using the same phrases when talking to my client. So for the Intro Run, and each time I do a Run, I would say:

"Okay, [name], *I'm just going to touch these points on the sides of your head. So now just be open to receive whatever you need to know, in whatever form it comes."*

This makes it clear that it is time for Penetrating Heaven, as distinct from Zero Balancing, and it implies that something is about to happen. I repeat this phrase each time I do a Run, so it becomes an anchor phrase that clients associate with altered state experiences. So, whenever I touch the points in future Runs and say these words, the client knows what is coming. This helps them to get into that state of mind more quickly and easily.

Eventually, when someone becomes a regular client, I no longer need to say anything when touching the points because they know the score, and they are already on their way.

So, to summarise: I find the points with a gentle, light touch and hold them with attention, applying one of my gears, until I sense working signs, which is when it is time to come off the points and release them. It is not necessary to tell the client that I am taking my hands away (not least because they often still feel my fingers on the points anyway). Their experience will usually have already started, and I don't want to interrupt it by talking.

Checking In: "How Are You Doing?"

After the Intro Run is a good opportunity to check in with the client, to ask how they are and what is happening. Getting the client's feedback helps me to address any obstacles that may inhibit their experience.

Bearing in mind that the Intro Run is just a short 2-minute taster to test the water, sometimes nothing will have happened yet. I want the client to know that this is okay - after all, it is early in the session. So that they stay open to the process, I may phrase my enquiry as follows: "Were you aware of anything happening?" or "Do you feel you are starting to get answers yet?"

If it is obvious from the working signs that the client is having a good journey experience, I may just silently carry on with the Zero Balancing Protocol without disturbing them, and I will check in with them for feedback later on. This way the process can continue.

Sometimes I may just tell the client: "That was the Intro Run. You may or may not have started to get answers, but I'm going to get on with the Zero Balancing bodywork now."

If the client feels that nothing has happened yet, then I reassure and remind them that more will happen as they relax more deeply and that they will get more as the session goes on.

For the later Runs I allow them more time, and with the added effect of the Zero Balancing clients can go into a very deep relaxed state. Because of this, my voice doesn't always bring them back straightaway, or sometimes they need a few moments to be able to reply. So before I check in with them, I will do a pass in their upper back to bring them back gently before speaking.

There is a chance that checking in will interrupt their experience. Therefore, after enquiring "How are you doing?", it is good to ask them "Would you like more time?" Then I can simply repeat the Run to take them back to where they left off.

In later Runs, if a client still isn't getting anything, then I may use other fulcrums. (See page 158-159)

The client can also easily lose track of time and feel like they have been gone for hours. I've had sessions where I checked in with the client after an early Run and asked them: "Okay, how was that?", only for them to take this as a signal that it was the end of the session!

Asking "How was that?" does sound rather final, whereas "How are you doing so far?" implies that we are only part of the way through the session and there is more to come. Also, for the later Runs, when checking in with the client, it is good to tell them how much time we have left and reassure them there is enough time for another Run, if they wish.

Naturally, responses vary between clients, so checking in gives very individual feedback. One client said she had received so many ideas that she was afraid of forgetting something. She had been lying there making a mental list, desperately trying to remember it all, so she suggested that I have a pen and paper ready to take dictation for her!

In practice I haven't needed to do this with anyone else, although soon afterwards another client asked if she could make her own notes during the session. I doubted if she could switch between journeying and writing. But she would stop, ask for a pen and paper, sit up to write, and then lie back down to resume the session. This worked well for her.

Obstacles on the Path

Shamanic practitioners say that there are two types of fear when embarking on a vision quest: Some people are afraid of stillness, silence and solitude because of what they may find there. Others are afraid that nothing will happen, as if they are somehow not worthy or good enough for something to happen.

I found that clients who are afraid of what might happen will try to resist, i.e. they will try to control or block the experience. And clients who are afraid that Penetrating Heaven might not work for them will try too hard; they try to 'do it'. Both of these types of fear create a tension that can act as an obstacle to the experience. However, I hoped this would be eased by the relaxation afforded by the Zero Balancing Protocol.

Clients Trying To Resist

Some people are apprehensive and don't want to have something 'done to them', so they resist the experience and nothing happens. However, because they have successfully blocked their journey, they know that they can also stop it whenever they want to, so they feel in control. This allows them to trust and let go, and as a result they relax and receive more of an experience in later Runs or in future sessions.

Clients Trying Too Hard

Some people are anxious that Penetrating Heaven won't work for them, so they try too hard to get answers. They want to know how the process works, what to do and how to do it, when all they really need to do is relax and let go. Again, this becomes a lot easier in later Runs or in future sessions.

Nobody is going to choose a trivial question. It will be something that is important to them, and this creates tension. Anticipation of a 'result' brings with it the idea of 'success' and 'failure'.

Some clients doubt themselves and their intuition. They say: "I'm not very good at this sort of thing." Kate, for example, said: "I worry that I won't get anything" and "It's like being in school", with that old familiar pressure to get the answer right. I assured her there would be several Runs and she seemed relieved when I said: "Don't worry if you're not getting anything yet."

Some clients worry if they are doing it right, or in the right way, and wonder what is going to happen - or what is *supposed* to happen. So I explain to them that you don't have to do anything. There is no right or wrong experience, so just relax. You can't do this wrong!

Clients who feel the need to 'do' or 'make it happen', as opposed to letting it happen, ask if it is important for them to put their awareness in the points while I'm touching them. Zero Balancing brings mind and body together where we touch, and sometimes in a ZB session it can be helpful to ask the client to "put your mind where you feel my hands", although this is not necessary for Penetrating Heaven, unless their question happens to be about a particular part of their body. (See page 193-194)

I once read about a meditation technique where you place a penny coin on your Third Eye (between your eyebrows). The sensation of the coin draws your attention to this area. And when you remove the coin, you are still aware of the sensation of the coin being there, just as some clients feel my fingers still on the points even after I have taken my hands away. It is an interesting idea to not only put my mind into my fingers when I touch the points, but also to ask the client to put their attention where they feel my fingers, so that they 'meet me there' at interface. I discovered that some of my clients were doing this on their own anyway, and it worked for them. However, it is not necessary for the client to do this (and trying too hard can be counterproductive). They can just relax, let go and let me do the work.

Client Doubts: "Am I Just Making It Up?"

"Of course it's happening inside your head, Harry.
Why should that mean that it's not real?"
- Albus Dumbledore
(in the movie "Harry Potter and the Deathly Hallows")

When a client gets an answer to their question, it may not make sense to them at first, and they may doubt their experience of what happened or dismiss it as 'just my imagination'. This is when writing it down on a capture sheet can help to make sense of it later on.

Even when a client receives an answer that does make sense to them, they may say: "I am getting answers but I think I must be making it up!"

Sandra Ingerman, a teacher of Shamanism, says (on The Shift Network):
"Don't fight your mind, because your mind is going to tell you that you are making it up, because this is what you were conditioned to do by your family, teachers and society."
"To fight with your mind is a waste of time, and of your own journeys.
"If your mind is telling you 'I'm just making it up' then say 'I agree. Yes, I am making it up!' It frees us then."

Sometimes the 'random' images we receive may seem meaningless. But they must come from somewhere, from deep inside of us, and perhaps they make sense to us on a sub-conscious level.

If we are making it up, we may ask why are we making up this and not something else; and how else would it look if our Higher Self, or sub-conscious mind, communicated to us?

In the end the important thing is whether the experience was useful, whether the client feels that they have gained a new perspective or clarity, and whether they have received something meaningful.

Working With What Comes Up

Sometimes the answer comes quickly, or early on in the session. Then I encourage the client to ask further questions. For example, if their question was "What is stopping me...?" and they have already got the answer, their next question might be "What can I do about it?" or "What is my next step?" As you receive one piece of the puzzle, you can ask for the next.

Rona got her answer early but found it confusing, so I suggested she have another Run and ask for more clarity on that answer. We can work with what comes up in this way.

Maria said she didn't get anything. "Just some sadness came up." But when I asked her if that sadness could relate to her question in some way, she brightened up: "Oh yes!" So the client can interpret what they experience within the context of their framed question. One client said: "It's about connecting to yourself but it's also about connecting the dots."

Abby went into her session with a question that she wanted the answer to, but she was surprised to find that she actually needed to know something else first. The first thing to bubble up for her was that she needed to know that she still had some unresolved grief - it was as if her 'wisdom within' was prioritising what came up. It was only after she acknowledged this grief that she then received the answer to the question in her Frame. She said:

"*Sometimes we don't need more knowledge but we need to acknowledge more.*"

Getting Answers, and Client Feedback

"Extraordinary! - Gentle yet powerful, what comes up!"

At first clients may say they get "nothing", then they report seeing some "random images", lights and colours. But these are not just plain ordinary colours: "That was awesome. I have never seen such colours before!"

Then images start to flow and the client sees "pictures and symbols in [their] mind's eye", or perhaps memories or scenes that are meaningful to them or that confirm their intuitive feelings.

Images and symbols may seem random or irrelevant but they are the language of the sub-conscious mind, so they have meaning and can therefore have an effect on us. This can be a helpful suggestion to make to clients, to reassure them that what they receive may still be relevant.

"Imagination is more important than knowledge.
Imagination is the language of the soul. Pay attention to your imagination
and you will discover all you need to be fulfilled."
- Albert Einstein.

Answers can be symbolic or metaphorical rather than literal or in words. Sometimes our experience is open to interpretation, and we may not even have to find meaning in it. Maybe it is beyond meaning, but it offers confirmation that we are connected to something greater than ourselves.

"Mythological symbols touch and exhilarate centres of life beyond the
reach of vocabularies of reason and coercion."
- Joseph Campbell.

Usually, the symbols that the client receives do make intuitive sense and are meaningful:

"I found that my intuition was quite keen to communicate with me symbolically, and I did indeed feel that I was given greater clarity on areas of my life that are meaningful to me."

Some clients have described a stream of fast-moving images, "like looking out of a car window". One said it was "like a flick-book" of images one after the other, like watching a movie, but "too fast for it to be my imagination". It contained old childhood scenes and memories, in detail.

Some clients say that Penetrating Heaven not only gives them images but also the feeling that they are actually there in the scene and having a full multi-sensory experience, complete with smells, sounds and feelings:

"Wow, it really takes you places!" and "It is deep, and transports you to another realm!"

The images are clear and detailed: "You can't push it away or ignore it, it's undeniable", and the experience is evidently more profound than just random, dreamy imaginings.

"If I try to remember or recreate the images, then the image is diluted and not as vivid."

"I can't reproduce that by myself, by daydreaming, imagination or 'trying to' do it."

.....

"Your work is truly magic!"

"Lots of insights - all completely effortless!"

Journeys are not always a visual experience. Some people receive sensations, or hear words spoken. Sometimes the answer seems so simple that it is easily dismissed at first, for example: "Let go." But it can be persistent. One client said that a particular word kept coming up for her that was relevant to her question. Another told me: "Answers came in the form of a dialogue", a full conversation. Some people speak of "downloading stuff" - useful, practical information.

Sometimes getting answers requires more than one Run, and a bit more relaxing Zero Balancing bodywork. Once, after the Intro Run, I asked my client: "Do you feel that you have started to get answers yet?" And they replied: "No, just more questions!" and "It's just opened up a can of worms!" After a later Run I enquired: "How is your can of worms now?" And they laughed: "Yes, that's better!"

Sometimes clients get their answer quickly, so they ask another question. Some even begin the session with more than one question in mind and receive answers to each one:

"Questions were indeed answered, and sometimes the question I was going to ask next!"

Some clients experience the retrieval of long forgotten memories or emotions that are relevant to their question. This may be a cue to acknowledge or forgive something.

Other clients get a "shift of perception", "a new perspective" or "realisations about [their] issue". It is also common for clients to feed back that they received "confirmation" and "clarity" on big decisions.

Some people tell me that the answer 'popped into their head', while others say that their answer 'arose': "It bubbled up from a place within me, rather than popping into my head."

A few clients have doubted if their answer really came from within, and they insisted that it was instead something from outside of them coming in. So the jury is still out on whether it is the client who is penetrating Heaven, or whether it is Heaven that is penetrating the client.

Sometimes the answer to the question comes not from within the person but occurs 'outside', in the world around them. For example, they find meaning or relevance in the call of a seagull as it flies past the window, or in the screech of brakes in the street outside just at a key moment in the session.

S.J. had a vision of someone letting go of a balloon. This may not have made sense at first, but afterwards, as she left the session, she actually saw a little girl letting go of a balloon. And then later, while viewing social media, she saw a tribute video to a close friend who had died, and in the video, again, was an image of someone letting go of a balloon.

Coincidence? Possibly, but perhaps the coincidences and synchronicities that occur during a session are meaningful because they take place in a different realm or state of consciousness - one where these things are significant. It is up to the client to decide what they make of it, or whether it has meaning. But these occurrences often suggest a glimpse of something beyond our everyday life, a connection to something greater than us, reaffirming our place in the world.

.....

"Thank you so much, that was truly amazing."

Bodywork for the Mind

There are many ways to access altered states of consciousness: meditation, sound, breath-work, or even drugs. But with Zero Balancing, the experience of the mind is anchored in the physical body because structure and energy are balanced simultaneously.

"My session with Gethyn was wonderfully relaxing. When he touched my head, it was like a 'hotline' to the universe, and I felt connected to an inner wisdom that meant my intuition was able to offer guidance and a deep state of peace and joy. The bodywork complimented this beautifully, and there was a congruence between mind, body and spirit."
- Sharon

People instinctively appreciate the combination of bodywork with altered states of mind because it truly embraces all of us. The experience is fully grounded, and we can feel it.

"Zero Balancing is a very relaxing and grounding treatment, which reminds me a little of Cranio-Sacral Therapy. I found it allowed a deeper sense of letting go in my body compared to many other treatments I've tried. Penetrating Heaven also encouraged a deep 'dropping' into myself, allowing for clarity and insights to arise. Gethyn explained the process clearly and held the space very well. He has a very calm and nurturing energy, allowing me to feel safe and supported throughout. I found the session a useful experience for some much needed me-time and for deeper clarity about issues I was facing in my life."
- Hannah

Zero Balancing touches the most physical part of us, our bones, yet it can have a very profound effect on the non-physical part of us, our mind. This adds an extra dimension.

"I did not expect it to actually work because I have previously attended a hypnosis session at the University of Sussex and I found out I am not very suggestible. However, during the Penetrating Heaven technique I immediately felt the touch to be kind of full of energy... One after another,

words started to pop up that seemed very relevant to my question... I have to say it was a very profound inner experience, probably more profound than any other inner experience I have achieved either through introspection or substances."
- Nora

With Zero Balancing, the session is anchored in the physical body, in our bones, so we literally embody our experience and integrate it into our being. And because of this, the transformative experiences that occur from the altered states stay with us. It is not unusual for clients to recount a session even years later and still feel moved by it.

"The images that come are really vivid and memorable, so they truly 'live' in you. I still remember my inner visions from the first session you gave me. In fact, I don't think they will ever leave me."
- Gabriele

As I offered Penetrating Heaven to a wider audience, more and more people began to liken it to shamanic work they had experienced, and felt a transformative healing quality: "The last time I felt like this was after shamanic healing." Another client even described Penetrating Heaven as "like shamanic journeying without all the fuss and drumming!"

"The session was quietly shamanic, and physically grounding. It helped me to focus my awareness towards a question that is important to me, and to relax in a way that allowed me to receive answers from different levels of my psyche. Gethyn was sensitive, and held the space very well. The quality of quiet that I experienced during the session was beautiful. I left feeling rested, more deeply connected with myself, and with some useful food for thought. I would recommend Gethyn's treatments highly. Thank you!"
- Hannah-Rose

Responses: Common Themes

Everybody is different and each individual experience is unique. However, from feedback I did notice some common themes that seem to occur quite frequently. These are:

- Ancestral journeys, childhood memories and past lives
- Encounters with spirit guides, angels or animal totems
- Journeys out of the body
- Journeys inside the body, or an experience of surgery

I do not try to steer the client's journey in any particular direction. I only list the common themes here in an effort to make sense of them and what they may mean.

Ancestral Journeys, Roots or Past Lives

Zero Balancing touches the energy of bone, and many different cultures make a connection between our bones and our ancestors, including Chinese Medicine and African healing. As John Lockley, a South African sangoma, says in his book "Leopard Warrior":

"Our flesh rests on our bones. To connect with our soul, we need to connect deeply with our bones. As a tree connects with its roots and reaches deep into the earth, so human beings have a responsibility to connect with their bones, and our bones are a living embodiment of our ancestry and ancestors. Hence, in the isiXhosa and isiZulu languages the word for bones (amathambo) is also used in reference to ancestors. It is often said that if people want to understand their life path, it is a good idea for them to remember their childhood and their natural tendencies and gifts. Understanding where we come from and developing a relationship with our ancestors is the next level to greater spiritual emancipation."

In Penetrating Heaven many clients have the experience of going back to visit scenes from their childhood. These may be old memories coming up, complete with the emotions associated with them, but they can feel like "more than just a memory". Sometimes people say that their visual movie of childhood scenes was like a whole new experience in old, familiar childhood settings.

Some people feel that the purpose of their experience of going back to childhood scenes was to show them or remind them of who they really are - to reconnect them with their true nature that started to blossom in their childhood innocence, before it was repressed or put aside.

Traditional cultures acknowledge their ancestors and their origins, honouring the very blood in their veins. They sing songs or dance or tell stories to remind them of who they are and where they come from, to connect to their roots, that their lives may bear fruit. It is an important part of our identity that is perhaps missing in modern life when people settle further from home, either migrating by choice or becoming displaced by circumstances beyond their control.

An Italian woman who had lived in England for many years framed her question around where to live, now that her children had left home. She saw images of her Italian ancestry, old photos of different generations of her family, and revisited her old childhood home. Some time afterwards she moved back to Italy.

Another woman told of her experience of walking up the hill to her ancestral family home, where she met her dad and her uncle but "as boys dressed in scruffy clothes" from before her time. Yet she still knew who they were, then they all walked along the road together.

B. reported being at the family farm with her cousins, but in her grandmother and grandfather's time. It was as it was then, and it was like she was there. Granny shouted at them for being noisy because Grandad was ill in bed (they had been to visit him). This was a real actual memory, and she saw "the black hearth, the under-stairs pantry, the stuffed pine marten in the glass case on the landing, the mounting block outside, the curved steps outside" in every detail.

M. described a slide show or "flick book" journey, revisiting scenes from her childhood, "things I've seen and done", especially with her cousin, who was then dying with cancer. She also had an experience of flying, mentioning a ride she had once taken in a helicopter over the countryside where she grew up: "I'm flying over all the places I saw when I was in the helicopter - but I'm not in a helicopter!"

"Every time I have a session, at first I think nothing is happening but gradually I seem to drift back to my childhood. Then I get lots of pictures in my mind in quick succession, rather like flicking through the pages of a book - but not too fast, so I can enjoy them. It feels like I'm really there again, not just remembering, because my memory has been jogged by the pictures. One thing I have realised is that I'm always happy and nearly always outdoors, except for being in the carpenter's shop, playing in the sawdust and shavings pile or in the granary at the farm. (It wasn't like a movie, it was real. I was really there. I could even smell the wheat and the wood shavings.) I'm never in school, which was dreary and uninspiring, or in church (dreary again!) Also, I'm never sad like when Dad died or when I was ill. These are the pictures I remember best: Walking to school and finding bird nests, lizards, lambs in the fields. Finding plants I hadn't seen before. Walking up the lane noticing the details, moss, rocks, flowers. Up at the farm in the hay (I could smell the hay), riding ponies with my cousin. Going for Sunday morning walks with Dad to the pool and catching minnows in a jam jar, then releasing them. Watching a mother mallard with all her babies riding on her back. Everything to do with nature, I suppose, and being free and outside."

These childhood experiences seem to be more than mere memories or flights of fancy. They tend to focus in on particular aspects of what is important to the person - revealing our "natural tendencies and gifts", as John Lockley says - and on what we feel a deep connection to.

Elizabeth saw herself in the chapel of her childhood village. There was a funeral service for a local man, Walter. A neighbour spoke to the congregation and asked if anyone else wanted to say anything. To her surprise, although nervous, Elizabeth stepped up and said a few words about her childhood with Walter and his prized dog, Chum. She told me that when Walter had left school to work, he had to give his dog to her family, and she had felt bad about it. Walter is still alive, so perhaps this 'funeral' was a symbolic laying to rest of these feelings.

Some clients have had a sense that this type of experience touches on ancestral healing. Others interpreted their experience as being deeply held memories belonging to past lives.

Karen's question was about her financial situation: "Why am I only surviving instead of thriving?" During the session she saw what she believed to be her past lives going way back in history, showing poverty and hard times. She felt it was in answer to why she was still only surviving in her present life, unable to break that pattern and thrive as she felt she should.

Encounters

Traditional shamanism can involve journeys beyond time and space to non-ordinary reality or invisible realms to find a teacher or guide, and ask them for help with a particular quest. They may appear in the form of an animal, a mythical figure or an ancestor.

Some of my Penetrating Heaven clients have had encounters with other beings or guides:

Claire saw people, who she thought were therapists of some kind, working in the dark, although there was light "like during an eclipse". And there was dialogue, i.e. questions and answers. When I asked if this dialogue made sense, her answer was an emphatic: "Yes!"

Alain said he met a group of other beings who spoke to him in French (his native tongue), which he found unusual because "I don't dream or think in French anymore". They were grouped around him, "like being surrounded by surgeons on an operating table". Then they turned to stone, like standing stones. Another figure came and took Alain flying through the sky. He was shown planet Earth and told that there is more work for him to do here.

.....

Encounters With Animals

Sometimes clients have an encounter with a particular animal that helps to answer their question, or they feel it is their spirit animal, animal totem or a spirit guide in animal form.

Claire had the experience of a powerful black panther. She said she was following in its paw prints, and then she really felt she was walking in its paws. She experienced the sensitivity, the groundedness and the awareness - and she got answers to her questions.

Sometimes the encounter may be with more than one animal. As one client reported: “There was a bizarre menagerie of lots of different animals.”

Marie showed some obvious working signs in her first session. She started turning her head from side to side, her body twisting and writhing. She arched her back off my massage table, then bared her teeth and growled, followed by the occasional happy laugh like it was fun. At the end of the session she sat up and said: “Wow, it’s a lot like journeying isn’t it?” Then I asked: “Did you go anywhere nice?” She smiled: “Oh yes, there were lots of animals!”

Jacqui saw a cobra and felt that she, too, was a cobra, “like the yoga pose”, so that her legs were the snake’s body and tail, firmly rooted on the ground, solid, but the rest of her body was upright, erect, alert. She felt as if she had been “called” to be visible and present.

Beth had an experience of talking to birds - a buzzard, a kingfisher and a woodpecker - and having conversations with them, asking questions about their life and getting answers: “[The bird] was talking to me, telling me about its life!” While lying on my massage table, she was given a buzzard’s perspective of how humans in aircraft “trespass” in their skies, and she relayed details of the bird’s diet, nesting habits, number of eggs, even the incubation time. These were all specific and accurate, as I checked afterwards. I wondered if it was possible that she had read all this information in a book but she said that if she had read it somewhere, then it had not been recently. It was so fluent and unhesitating that even if she had remembered it all from some time ago, it was still a stunningly accurate memory retrieval, if not a full communication download.

Encounters With Angels

One day I had a new client come for Zero Balancing, who had read about it in an article in "Kindred Spirit" magazine. During the session I included Penetrating Heaven and she said it felt like healing. She revealed that she was a healer and she practised a type of healing called Belvaspata. In it, she doesn't touch the client but calls in the angels to work with the person instead while she 'gets out of the way'.

The following day a regular client came for a session, having just heard the news that her father had suffered a stroke earlier that morning. It was a shock for her but she still wanted to go ahead with the session. My own dad was recovering from a stroke, too, so my heart went out to her.

As I started to do Penetrating Heaven, I suddenly wondered whether, in light of her news, it was really appropriate for her to have a journey experience, and I began to hesitate as I thought about my own dad.

I had never worked with angels before, but as I held the points I decided to try asking the angels to come and help. Then I took my hands away and I sat well back in my chair in order to get out of the way.

I did very little work on the client after that, and at the end of the session she smiled and said: "I felt like I was being held by angels." (I had not told her.) Thankfully her dad made a quick recovery and was discharged from hospital the following day.

The next day I got a call from a new client wanting to book a session of Zero Balancing, and her name was... Angelika!

Angels were never really my thing and I had never tried working with them before that day. At the time I was focused on developing my Penetrating Heaven technique and wanted to prove that it works on its own, without any outside help from angels, thank you! And so this is not something that I pursued or even intended to include in this book.

However, since that day, so many clients have mentioned angels or an angelic presence as part of their session experience that I have been unable to ignore it. After all, my technique is called "Penetrating Heaven" and Heaven is where angels are said to come from, bringing messages to us here. So far, however, such angelic encounters have eluded me personally. I just work here!

M.R. (Session 7)

"The journey was me lifting off, dancing in air (not in the room - in another space) surrounded by angels. Then I saw a child safely and happily asleep in a bed. I withdrew to see where they were and there were many children in bed in a long room, looked over by an initially fearsome looking being but on closer inspection, a protector. This is in regard to the question of my relationship, as we are considering adoption. It is something we both want to do but are also scared of doing. So the journey was important. Then I was whisked away to a place of light, and walking down from a sort of podium or building was my guide. He gave me advice which was specific and will, I am sure, prove to be important also."

Encounters With Family

Lisa had been having problems with her family dynamics. She said her session created a healing circle for all of them:

"… I explained to you after the incredible experience that I saw an angel above Earth, and I became the angel and flew down to my brother's house. My brother has Asperger's and lots of mental health problems associated with that, because of our emotionally neglectful upbringing with parents who knew no better due to their own experiences and because it has also transpired that my dad has Asperger's (undiagnosed but all traits are there, same as my brother). He often cuts me off from his life unexpectedly over a menial grudge and lately it's been his record of 1.5 years of no contact. My session with you involved me as an angel, first throwing cluster bombs of stars around him to draw his attention to my presence, followed by me swirling stars around his heart and around his head and then swirling them around him in a cyclone. After some time doing that, I raised him up above earth with me and brought in my parents and got them to hold hands. I conducted a ceremony in which I facilitated them all looking at each other with compassion, love, forgiveness and understanding. They moved in a circular motion/dance looking at each other with loving kindness and peaceful connected unity. I continued to swirl stars around them. I brought in my daughter (a bright and conscious spark) and my nephew (on the autistic spectrum) and continued to facilitate, getting my family members to celebrate the children's beautiful existence and their contribution as the next generation, and to send unconditional love and acceptance and bathe in the joy of their purity and innocence. The whole ceremony felt deeply healing and joyful, and my role was to bring unity to their disconnection and lack of love (that has always been apparent) through my guidance and just soooo many sparkles of stars. This continued for my whole session and I finished it by thanking them all for their time.

After the session I went to [a café]. I ordered food, and it took me almost an hour to return back to the earth plane in a fully functioning way. The food really helped to ground me.

Since that time, I have had the odd message - Happy Christmas, and Happy New Year from my brother - which is not a lot, but still quite a breakthrough compared to how things have been with his communication. I spent time with my parents both Christmas Day and Boxing Day, and both my parents were hugely joyful. My mum, who is usually quite reserved and bitter, even got up to sing and dance! I've never in my life seen her do that! WOW!

I was already on a path to healing family and ancestral pain over recent years, particularly this year. I have journeyed deep with gong baths and other meditations and body work, and what I experienced with you was like a beautiful icing on the cake I've been baking lately.

I feel really at peace in myself for the first time in my life, with the combined work in recent months. I've had so much sadness and pain for most of my life from taking on board so much trauma from my childhood and the continued adult relations with my family. I've felt different from the moment I was born. I have memories of questioning why I am with 'this family' from a young age and wishing that my true family from the universe would save me from the pain. As I age, I realise more and more my important role within this earth family I was born into and from my heart know that I am giving something different to my daughter. I realise that all the pain I've felt, and how I've healed and grown against all the adversity, has brought me a special gift that I can share with others. Thank you for facilitating me to journey deep in angelic realms and take my family there."

Journeys Out of the Body

In one of the earliest experimental sessions, Mike had an out-of-the-body experience. Other clients have had journeys out of their body or experienced astral travel, but this was usually something that they had experienced before and they were used to doing it, so it wasn't alarming to them.

Claire also reported looking down on her body lying on my massage table and seeing me sitting behind her, at her head.

Jane said she was looking down on herself, not on the massage table in real time, but having a birds-eye view of her day up until the session: "It looks so absurd, rushing about, worrying about being late or how I look." She felt amused "as a detached observer":

"Being a regular meditator and feeling safe, I was able to relax into the session straight away, and experienced a deep level of drifting, feeling as if the walls had been removed from the edges of my experience. I very quickly felt a very different perspective, as if I could look down on the events of my life, of that morning, in a kind of custodial way, with amusement and in a detached way. This gave me a reassuring feeling, as if there is nothing to worry about. That feeling has stayed with me on and off during the week, along with the feeling of detached amusement. This level of reassurance is very helpful, allowing me to step away from concerns and see them in a different light. It feels like tapping into my higher self, or greatness, leaving behind small habits and concerns."

Nancy felt and saw herself "emerging from a cocoon, and lots of old stuff was falling away". This was accompanied by memories of her past self.

Journeying Inside Your Own Body

As well as having the experience or perspective of traveling outside of their physical body, some clients have reported going inside their own physical body and journeying within. This gave me the idea for clients to frame their question around their health and explore their symptoms, which was to be a further development of Penetrating Heaven. (See pages 187-199)

Claire's frame was that she was seeking more balance in her life. First of all, she saw a pair of brass weighing scales in front of her. Then she saw a white light, but she 'jumped' and pulled back as she felt herself floating, disorientated, not knowing where she was or if I was still there. She also felt herself being pulled to her right side into the dark (but not unpleasant). In her final Run she felt her eyes turn around in her head to face inside. Her eyes were seeing inside her. She could see the colour of her flesh and the individual blood vessels in detail. Then she saw a red bloody ball, and she was holding it in her hands. She said she had seen this before in a different therapy session and she hadn't known what to do with it, but this time she knew, and she just dropped it and let it go: "I don't need this anymore." Perhaps this act of letting go of what she no longer needed helped her to 'balance the scales'.

Psychic Surgery

Some sessions brought up a theme of surgery, with clients either feeling at the end of the session as if they had just had surgery, or feeling like they were actually having surgery performed on them during the session.

At the end of her first session, Sarah told me she felt like she was "in post-op, on a slab". Another client said she felt that she had been "split down the middle". These descriptions may sound gruesome but they were not unpleasant and ultimately very liberating.

Karen had a good Intro Run. Then, as I continued the ZB Protocol in her lower back and legs, she thought I was touching her head. She felt a brief pain in her right ankle which "released something" and the HMV at the feet was "really helpful, it felt like I was opened up".

Later on, I took my hands away and sat well back in my chair to allow her a long Run. During this time Karen's body moved around on the table, twitching. And she later said her left leg felt as if it had been locked in place; she couldn't lift it but could shake and twist it.

Karen said the left side of her body went cold (she identified this as a spiritual presence), and there was a sense that she was being operated on. Blockages were being removed, some unseen beings were doing surgery on her, "drilling into the left side of my temple", and there was a sense of "stuff being pulled out" (as far as I could tell the experience was painless!) Finally she saw "white healing light coming through my crown, flooding my whole body".

The Plateau: A Natural Pause

Although there seems to be no limit to what people can experience, the expanded states of consciousness and the journey experiences cannot be sustained indefinitely. There is a limit to how much we can do in one session, even if we have plenty of time. As you may remember, earlier in the book I described how I once did an experimental session with a friend where we had all afternoon free to explore, but after several productive Runs the session then reached a plateau and came to a natural close.

Usually, by the third Run, the client will have received their answer, and got what they came for. When I check in with them, they tell me that nothing new is happening, "just more of the same, really". They are not able to go any further, and the effect is beginning to level off.

At first I thought this meant that the effect was stalling and that therefore it needed to be reinforced by touching the points again. However, many people feel that this plateau is an important part of the session. One client told me: "Sometimes when the question has been answered, then it gives way to healing relaxation." Other clients agree that they drop into a deep, healing space ("the most relaxed I've ever felt in my life") for a period of digesting and processing the answer, which is an important part of the experience.

And so I sit back and allow the client to remain in this space, in the stillness, for the remainder of the session.

Many of my clients agree: "[First] the answers come through and then healing comes through." One client felt that the healing was coming from the same place as her answer: her Higher Self.

Closing the Session

I try to end each session with a good long final Run and then check in with the client to make sure they are ready to finish. I found that it's best to do a pass in the upper back first to gently bring the client back into the physical before I speak to them. Usually they will have gone into a very deep place, so they need a little time before they can talk to me.

I also found that it's good to explain to them that I haven't quite finished yet because some people take the sound of my voice as a cue to get up off the massage table. So I say that I am just going to do a bit more Zero Balancing to bring them back into their physical body, and that I will work my way down to their feet to close the session.

Then all that remains is for me to complete the Closing Sequence of the ZB Protocol.

The Closing Sequence is a 'cascade' of Half Moon Vectors from the head down to the feet. The final HMV at the feet serves as a good cue for the client that the session is complete.

The Peruvian shaman don Oscar Miro-Quesada talks the client back into their body, and back into the physical realm, by telling them: "*Be aware of your breath, be aware of your body, the table you are on, the room you are in...*"

Some clients who have experienced forms of shamanic journeying that do not involve any physical touch have found the Closing Sequence to be very welcome, and they tell me that my holding their feet at the end has a grounding effect, so they feel 'back in their body'.

Having finished the ZB Protocol, I address the client by name to tell them that I have finished but I assure them that there is no hurry and suggest that they may like to have a stretch before they get up. Then I wait for the client to roll over to one side and sit up before I ask them how the session was for them.

When I was researching Penetrating Heaven and eagerly awaiting feedback, I had to learn to be patient and resist the urge to ask the client too many questions at once. I wanted to know what had happened, whether they had received their answer, whether it was useful, and whether their experience was visual, auditory or kinaesthetic. But of course it was important to give the client time!

At the end of the session I provide the client with a capture sheet and encourage them to write down their experience while it is still fresh in their mind. This serves to solidify the memory so that they don't forget any important details.

Some people may write a full account while others just note down the key bullet points. Some will do doodles or drawings because their experience was difficult to put into words. However, I encourage everyone to capture something of the session, even if it doesn't make sense, because it may make sense later on, sometimes even in the days that follow.

I also reassure the client that whatever they write down is private and that they don't need to show it to me or share it with me. The capture sheet is for them to take home with them, even if they don't look at it again. Just the act of writing or drawing something can help the person to process what happened.

Capturing the Vision

In the early days of experimental sessions, Mike would give me verbal feedback of his experiences. But sometimes it was easier for him to draw it rather than trying to put it into words.

Later on, more clients felt the need to draw or write things down at the end of the session. After her first session, my friend Mariella felt this was an important process and she strongly suggested that I make it part of the session for every client in order to help them capture the vision.

So at the beginning of the session, after framing their question, I show the client that there will be a capture sheet waiting for them at the end so that they can write down their answer.

And at the end of the session, I encourage the client to write down their experience of what happened and the answers they received, even if it is only in bullet points or doodles, and even if it doesn't make sense, in order to capture their inner journey while it is still fresh in their mind, so that they don't forget it, or start to doubt themselves and dismiss it later on.

People have told me that writing it down or drawing it helps them to capture their experience, which helps them to remember it, process what happened, and gain more clarity from it, because it can take time to digest. (As I said earlier, even if some of it doesn't make sense at first, perhaps it will make more sense a few days later.) Many clients have told me that Penetrating Heaven continues to work for several days afterwards and more insights continue to unfold. Some have sent me written accounts, drawings or paintings that they felt moved to produce at home after their session.

While people find it useful to write or draw their experience immediately after the session, a few clients have felt moved to get up off the massage table during a session and physically act out or perform what they had seen, felt or experienced, capturing and processing it in this way.

As don Oscar Miro-Quesada advises after a guided meditation (on The Shift Network):

"I encourage you to paint, draw, sculpt, write, bake, dance, cook, garden... Give some physical form to whatever inner experience you have been graced by."

In other words, give expression to the experience and bring it into the physical. As Miro-Quesada goes on to say:

"In this way... we allow all visionary encounters to have a pragmatic earthly service function. It becomes art, and art shall transform our world... May you carry this journey into your life."

And besides, as the dream teacher Robert Moss, creator of Active Dreaming, says: "*Souvenirs and mementos are nice to have.*" So just jot down or sketch something!

Answers may come directly or symbolically, for example as images or metaphors. These can be open to interpretation by the client but generally we can assume that the experience will relate directly to the client's framed question and intention in some way. And it is up to the client to make the connections in the context of their question, and to decide whether what they have received is useful or not.

Trust and Privacy

It is my belief that Zero Balancing opens us up and creates a space in which we can have experiences that are not ordinarily available to us. Through the deep relaxation achieved in Zero Balancing we can gain inspiration, insights and guidance, and also receive healing. So, Zero Balancing opens us up, and then Penetrating Heaven can help to create the focus and direction for the experiences that Zero Balancing enables us to have.

The client's experience relates to the individual's frame and question, or what is going on in their life. It also seems to depend on factors such as:

- how the client is in themselves, 'where they are at'
- their Donkey's willingness to let go and explore, and
- the person's belief system

Naturally, the way clients feed back their experience is their interpretation of what happened, and so they will couch it in terms that they recognise and relate to. It is personal to them.

At the end of a pure Zero Balancing session, the client will often have a relaxed smile. And after a session with Penetrating Heaven, the client will often have a quizzical expression and they ask me: "How much of that did you see?" or "Could you see what was happening?"

No, I don't see or share in what the client is experiencing. It is their own private experience. This privacy aspect helps the client to feel safe and builds trust in the whole process, which supports the good Donkey Connection. I don't need to know and they don't need to tell me. I say to them: "You don't have to tell me your question, and you don't have to tell me your answer."

For many clients this is a relief and a big advantage because naturally the questions they choose for the Frame are often deeply personal, and therefore they may not feel comfortable sharing them.

This aspect of Penetrating Heaven affords clients a level of privacy that some feel is lacking in other therapies. Some of my clients have told me of experiences with other therapies where they felt exposed and "at the mercy" of the therapist, and they have felt compromised because the therapist knows their 'stuff'.

With Zero Balancing and Penetrating Heaven, I don't need to know my client's 'stuff', neither their question nor their answer. This makes the process empowering for the client because I don't give them the answer; they receive the answer for themselves.

One client summed it up by saying that this level of privacy makes Penetrating Heaven a "sacred" experience.

Privacy helps the client, and it also helps me. The fact that I don't know what is happening enables me to stay emotionally detached, which helps me to get out of the way and hold the space, and allow whatever is happening to happen. All I do is to facilitate the client's experience, and this frees me up. Sometimes my clients' experiences have been profound, personal and emotional, so it was better that I didn't know what was going on until I received the feedback afterwards.

Even when clients are happy to share their experience with me, it may be difficult for them to express or put into words. For this reason, detailed feedback was sometimes hard to come by. At the end of a session, besides encouraging the client to write down what happened for them, I note down any verbal feedback they give me. Sometimes clients have also chosen to email me several days later with a fuller account of their experience.

I would like to thank the people who have shared their experiences with me for this book. In the following pages I will present some first hand accounts of my clients' experiences.

Case Examples

Altered states of consciousness allow us an opportunity to see things in a different way and open us up to new perspectives, giving clarity, understanding and even practical help:

Christine, an artist, was struggling with a sculpture she was working on. She felt stuck, so her Frame was for more ideas and inspiration for this piece. During the session she saw her sculpture but she was viewing it coming from the inside of the stone outwards, rather than the usual way of working from the outside in! She talked through the process as she lay on the massage table, working it out for herself, as I held the space.

Another artist, B.W., was struggling with a half-finished painting, so she framed the session around her work. During the session she said she could see her finished painting and then she could see how she had done it! Soon after this session she completed the painting.

.....

M.G. (Session 1)

M.G. was on the brink of emigrating from England to the USA. His questions concerned this move, his future career and the relationship with his American partner, who is a recovering alcoholic. In the Intro Run he saw the space shuttle at Cape Canaveral with the US flag, and saw this as a call to adventure. He later saw heroic and mythical figures, "like a movie clip", and then the city of Atlantis. He mentioned that he had recently had dreams about water, more specifically about drowning and being helpless, but this was now a feeling of having power over water. M.G. asked about his relationship and saw images of casinos and pulling down the lever on a one-armed bandit. He said he hates gambling and interpreted these images to mean that his relationship is a risk and he was eventually going to lose in the end.

E.B. (Session 1)

This client had recently qualified in Reflexology, and she was fortunate enough to be taking over another Reflexologist's practice. Her question was naturally about her future career. In her session she saw a vision of a peacock with its colourful feathers proudly on display. She interpreted this to mean that it is time for her to get noticed and to market her new practice. Then she saw herself running behind a horse-drawn wagon and she jumped on the back. (She saw this as riding on the back of the other Reflexologist's practice.) Then she saw a warm, bright fire to her left then a big oak door opened in front of her and it was time to step through it.

.....

N.A. (Session 2)

"It was more difficult this time to get into a place where I got answers. In the beginning I was feeling quite distracted and I was waiting for answers, and it seemed like I was generating them myself. However, when you touched my feet, I started to get lots of visual memories of me and my ex-partner. Then when you touched points on my neck and head, I started to get memories about his childhood, the hardships he went through in life, his loneliness and lack of connection to life. Then it somehow connected to my childhood and some of the things my parents experienced. Then I started to develop this intense feeling of emotional pain and compassion towards my ex-partner and all the things he had to go through in his life, and then tears started rolling down and my eyes began twitching again a lot. When I was feeling this intense sadness, I felt these words very clearly that were coming [from] somewhere outside of me that said "You helped him." These words were reassuring and they created a feeling of lightness. It felt like I was fighting these words, though, and I had a lump in my throat. I felt like it isn't fair that people go through suffering in life to learn things. But then I felt these words. "You don't know everything, you don't know the whole picture. You don't know why." After the session I cried and it felt liberating. I don't fully understand how this happened but I felt like I connected to some part that knows about the purpose of events and situations, and it seemed like every interaction and event that happens is there for a reason."

D.T. (Session 1)

D.T., a business woman, had recently split from her male partner. She had been reading about how the male and female principles are present throughout nature - for example, in an atom there are protons and electrons, i.e. positive and negative charges.

Her question or intention for the session was to explore the role of the masculine and feminine energies in her life, and about moving towards engaging her masculine energies.

The Intro Run resulted in D.T. having a personal realization that she had always looked outside of herself for the masculine to complete her. In her childhood she would escape her dysfunctional family by reading or watching movies, which all featured the female finding the male outside of herself, and being rescued. She realised that she had been neglecting her masculine side, and seeking it outside of herself. She understood that, if her masculine energy is weak or unacknowledged, then a stronger male energy from outside will dominate her.

From the second Run:
"I asked myself the question: 'Why do I engage my masculine in some areas (house, car, business) but not in the most important areas, such as my personal creative goals?' And the answer was: Actually throughout all areas it is only half engaged, if I'm honest! So I got lots of realizations, including the goal of balance between masculine and feminine, looking at past generations and seeing the pendulum swing from one extreme to the other in my mother, grandmother, and further back. One compensated the other. That's why balance is so important to rise above the swing..."

D.T. left her session with a sense that meditation can help to align these elements within - the physical, mental and emotional - and that this alignment can then play out in her life.

.....

G.T. (Session 1)

The following session combined the awareness of the physical body offered by Zero Balancing with the guidance and confirmation of the client's own personal path offered by Penetrating Heaven. It serves as a reminder that the answers are within us and we must take responsibility for what happens:

"This was my first ever session of Zero Balancing and Penetrating Heaven. You are encouraged to go into the work with a question that you would like guidance or clarity on, and personally I received an answer almost instantly. This then enabled me to pose further, related questions, so that a whole narrative unfolded for me.

Now 47, I have been interested in different modes of healing since my early 30s. Propelled by a personal history of illness and physical incapacitation, I have been on a search to tap ever more strongly into my own healing powers, both for myself and for others, and my initial question centred around what I could do to enhance my healing work. The very clear sense I got in reply was "Just keep doing what you're doing", accompanied by a really happy, positive feeling inside. Next I wanted to know: What's blocking or holding me back in developing my healing further?" "Nothing." Nothing is blocking me! I'm doing all the right things and the path is clear to keep growing. What a feeling of freedom, light and upliftment! I couldn't help myself and laughed with pure joy.

Gethyn proceeded to work on my body with ZB, which relaxed me down further, and then we had another go at PH. My original question answered, this time I enquired how I could make the effects of my healing work more profound on the physical level and received this: "By doing your own healing first." The ZB made me aware how much mental-emotional pain, some of it from long ago, I hold in my physical body, so it was clear what work I had to do. In order to shift a persistent core of "dark stuff" in the centre of my body, which I had often seen before and which I took to be old hurt and pain, I suddenly became aware that I had to work with my Third Eye. In a way, the Third Eye is a "button" I press to switch on the light which will chase away the darkness in my belly. Like Harry Potter waves his wand to invoke a Patronus Charm and blasts away the Dementors, if I switch on my inner light the darkness of pain will disappear. This confirmed that the path I'm already on is the right one.

Questioning further about what I needed to do to facilitate my healing work (both for myself and others; it is important to point out that, for me, the healing I do is never just for myself), I morphed into a Fire Angel who had an acute sense of right and wrong and who, with wrath and might, enforces healthy boundaries both within and without, and who works tirelessly for the light. As I felt my power and magnitude as the Fire Angel, I got a sense that there was someone standing behind me, so I turned around – and got a start: Very much in contrast to the glorious Light I beheld in front of me, behind me there was darkness, out of which numerous pale, impoverished, starving people, trailing into the darkness, stared up at me with large, dark, imploring eyes, saying: "We're waiting to follow in your path. We're waiting for you to blaze a trail for us."

While on the one hand I know that my work is going to serve people, I'm also aware that I cannot let them enfranchise me for their needs. Firstly, I still have healing of my own to do, and secondly it is imperative that I keep focusing on my own inner self, both now and when the time comes to eventually make myself more available to others. I can guide and support people in their work but ***their work is their own****. They have to do it themselves and I cannot let them weigh on me and drain me, even though they may expect me to carry them and do their work for them, as people generally do. It would be very wrong to let myself be flattered or charmed into doing this and I cannot allow that to happen – both for my own sake and theirs. I was very grateful for that clear, strong warning and reminder.*

For me, PH has served as helpful and welcome validation that I am on the right path, doing the things that are right for me, aligned with my intentions and desires. In addition, it has brought me useful insights that will enhance my further development. In a way I feel that, with Penetrating Heaven, Gethyn is helping to birth and support each person's own personal path, which is immensely valuable and not generally offered by practitioners of physical approaches. I am very grateful for what I've taken away from the session."

F.G. (Session 1)

"I did not know what to expect from the session, but I just knew that it was going to be a relaxing experience. Gethyn gave me an introduction of his work and said that I can ask a question of particular concern I am facing in my life (i.e. love, finances, job etc.) or instead I can ask a more general question, for example 'What do I need to know'. Then during the session some images will come into my mind that might answer my question.

Everything sounded just perfect, and I couldn't wait to start because at that moment I was not feeling well, had constant headaches and was feeling stuck in my life. He started touching my head and pressing some of the points of my head, neck and back and I started relaxing. The first moments of the therapy probably were the most amazing and magical moments. I saw myself in a dark misty place surrounded by trees, but then I realised that it was a cemetery. Suddenly I saw like a light at the end of the road and I started walking towards the light. The next thing I felt was myself lying on a cradle, possibly in a hospital, because there were windows and the room was white. I felt like everything was new to me, I was feeling like a new born just feeling alive, no thoughts, no feelings, just being present and observing. This was very strange but an amazing experience that is hard to explain. Then I saw a somebody approaching, probably a woman who was looking at me, maybe my mom because she was looking at me very happy. This was a very touching moment, because I do not have pictures of myself as a baby, and this moment was so beautiful.

For the rest of the therapy I saw different passages of my life, like a movie that helped me to answer and understand some puzzles of my life. After the therapy I was feeling very relaxed and with a feeling of more happiness within myself. Since I had the therapy, lots of things have started happening in my life! I strongly recommend his work. At this stage I even find it hard to explain all of the experience, but you have to live it to understand it."

.....

F.G. (Session 2)

A few weeks later F.G. came for another session. She was having a stressful time at work. She said she felt slow at her job, and as a result she was under pressure from her boss.

In the Intro Run she saw a tree and it was 'opening'. She said: "There was the trunk and the rest was a brain. Then the sky opened and light came down, and then it closed again."

In the next Run she received the words:

"You are born perfect. You need do nothing. You have learned fears and you carry them."

F.G. had a realization that she is slow at her work because as a child she was made to do chores instead of going out to play with the other children. She resented this and so she always did the chores slowly, and this pattern of behaviour had continued into adulthood.

In the final Run she saw a Native American anointing her with oil, on her knees and body. Then she saw her grandmother who used to put roast tomatoes on the instep of her feet and the fleshy area between her thumb and index finger if she had a sore throat as a child. This was a very touching memory for her.

When I closed the session with a final HMV at her feet, she said she felt really strong. She could see chains around her legs, but now she saw these chains were breaking.

.....

A.K. (Session 1)

This client had an uneventful Intro Run. However, as I continued with the ZB Protocol, working on her sacrum, lower back and ribs, she had an emotional release. We took a pause, then I repeated another Run for her to get insight into what these emotions were about:

"The introduction to what was going to happen was good. It had prepared me well and set my expectations. It was clear from the beginning that the upper rib area was going to be important. When you touched it with your flat palms it felt particularly nice, I felt held, supported, really safe, even in the emotional aspect. I felt the way I had felt as a kid before I started to fear the world. I felt a huge relief, as if some heavy and draining responsibility had been temporarily lifted off of me. When you applied pressure to the specific points in that area, a big release of old emotions flooded me completely. It was very clearly old stuff, stuff I couldn't quite remember or put my finger on. It wasn't even clear why it was making me cry, there wasn't anything negative about what I was observing. There were snapshots from when I was 5 and spending time at my grandparents' place. I remembered the simplicity of that time, the unconditional acceptance I was receiving from them, like I just could do no wrong. I was myself and it felt like "myself" was exactly what they were after. They were very responsive to me and we were creating different situations together.

My question at the beginning of the session was around what I should/ would love to do for a career, what my vocation was, and also how that ties in with finding my soulmate and starting a relationship. Should I focus on finding my path first, so I attract the man who's attracted to the much more focused, passionate and secure version of me?

The answers I was getting, as a clear voice of my inner wisdom, were along the lines of "Think about what you loved back then. What did you love before you stopped being you?" Those questions released further emotions and it was impossible to hold back tears. When you were touching my head, I felt actual electricity running from your fingers. I struggled at first to receive anything other than a string of massively random, unrelated images. It was clear I wasn't going to get a straightforward answer to my questions. After releasing some more stuff and trying again, I saw myself leaving a house - my future house. There was a strong and loving structure I was leaving behind the door. And I was on my way to another strong and loving structure. The wisdom I got from this, as well as from other images (like looking at the garden at sunset with somebody at my side who knew and understood me), was that my answers are going to get revealed whilst I'm enjoying living my life, not before, in preparation for it. I have hit the wall on the amount of wisdom I can extract from my current situation, because I have never loved, or committed to anything or anyone. And that's when I'll finally know myself. I'll know what I love and how I want my life to be. It was a very revealing session. I have been struggling with not knowing what to focus on in my life for so many years, and the answer is so simple - on everything and anything that I love. Every single day. Thank you so much, that was very useful and it explains so much about why I haven't been getting anywhere with my current, safe approach. It's just too emotionally dry, it's noncommittal and untrusting. A huge learning. It definitely helped to keep releasing blockages and coming back to receiving the wisdom time after time. Whilst the images weren't initially logically connected, when I finally hit the spot with the main learning, all the little ones fell into place right next to it. In terms of 'means' of communication, there were images, mainly static but some of them dynamic, plus of course the voice of wisdom, actual words in my head."

So you don't need to know your life's purpose before you can then go out and live and love - you need to go out and live and love in order to find your life's purpose! (It will find you!)

.....

A.K. (Session 2)

Several weeks later A.K. returned for another session. Having previously explored what she would love to do as a career, this time her framed question was about a future relationship and what she needed to know in order to make it happen:

"First of all, there were the physical sensations. (I felt hungry = hungry for love!) It showed me yet again that I'm starved of affection, closeness and tenderness. It's very easy for me to forget about it, in my silly pursuit of so-called independence. Again, there were certain areas, particularly below my shoulder blades, that were particularly sensitive (in a good way), and when I was 'suspended' it gave me an incredible sense of relief. Like I was being held, not just literally. The feeling symbolised being supported, looked after and as if somebody was carrying my load with me. I was reminded of what it feels like, and that I'd very much welcome that in my life.

This second session seemed to be less about releasing things and more about 'populating' my consciousness with clear images of what I would love. Very much the kind of thing I need right now, seeing as all I do is very skillfully pretend I don't need or want anything or anyone.

I was seeing and feeling very relationship-y things. I saw myself with this guy (he was my friend D. but I'm choosing to treat it as a symbol of the 'strong and gentle' vibe that I like). There was me pulling him by the arm, in a playful, cheerful manner, towards a meadow full of flowers, so we could dance in it. It almost looked like an eHarmony commercial.

He was bringing out my open, carefree side. I was the 'cute instigator' and he was the rock and the stabilising influence, entertained by my randomness and my dynamic, expressive personality. He found it disarming, endearing. I was sort of a satellite, free to roam, enjoying his trust, but drawn to him and always ending up by his side.

I also got many glimpses of the feelings that the above scenario would bring. It made me realise that there is nothing quite like a deep, sovereign relationship and that that's the only thing that can bring out those feelings. It's a very unique connection, and I think that the frustration I've been feeling, about not being able to connect with people on a deep enough level, is partially because I have been denying the need for that deep connection with my soulmate, trying to find it elsewhere.

That's a pretty big discovery. I have been putting a great amount of pressure on other, 'smaller' relationships to fill that void. Knowing this now releases the inner resources to focus on the 'correct' vision, not a bunch of smaller, misplaced, substitute visions.

I've learned that I do want a deep relationship with my soulmate and it's not lame. It's the only way to feel the way I felt in those glimpses.

Another message I got was 'You need to nourish your heart outside of the relationship' and other messages about men being free to come and go. (Hello, free will!) So it's not my job to control him, but to become the version of myself I am happy with and proud of. There's no ensuring I won't ever get abandoned and I might as well get over it.

*The whole session has made me realise how much I'll be putting on the next guy I want a relationship with. So many unmet needs, seriously behind on intimacy, physically starved and emotionally needy. How about just loosening up a bit? I've been playing the 'Nobody touch me, nobody come close' game for way too long. Waiting for my one and only to finally meet all my needs, meanwhile walking around with a big 'F*ck off' sign on my forehead, afraid of my space being invaded and my sensitivities violated, acting either arrogant or shy. Done with it. I want to flirt, allow some men to partially fulfil my need for attention, allow them to come closer, be more proactive myself because that's just what I want. It's fun and it's natural – no point being embarrassed about having normal, womanly needs. Being held, looked after, pursued, adored. Bring it on.*

So I received a clear vision of what my perfect relationship would look and feel like, then I was shown how deprived I am of the basics, and then I realised what illusions I've been feeding myself, which need to go.

Thank you, definitely very useful.
(Sometimes it's better to sleep on it to get more clarification of the learnings!)"

.....

M.R. (Session 9)

After deciding that the best question was "What do I need to know?", and working with that for a while, one day a regular client chose to ask one of the 'big' questions: "Who am I?"

"Questions:
Who am I?
What should I be doing?
How can I help J. [girlfriend]?

First Run:
I see myself in spirit world, not after death but now, as a child. This is how I feel I am. I look up to a higher being (my guide) who exudes love, wisdom, comfort. They point towards J. (also now in spirit). She is at peace with herself, strong, wise, sitting in protection of many children (like a teacher). She is huge, the children are tiny.

A door opens / a space opens up - a giant enters - I become the giant - they are me.

I, now powerful, with knowledge, awareness, able to do anything, fly through a portal, with J. at my side, into many worlds / universes - we explore. I lead the way - it is easy, beautiful, magical, cosmic, infinite.

A feeling of great compassion arises - compassion towards the earthly realm - our world / universe. Through my desire / intention / prayer, thousands of gold lights of healing and love descend, fall into the earthly realm - it is easy to do this and I have an understanding of a circular meaningfulness - that this is how it is / should be / must be - the lights descend into earthly realm, that ascends as a result and becomes spirit world that fuels source of everything / God.

In looking to the source of these gold lights, I see / know / feel their source - and enter or it enters me - a state of pure bliss. I reside here and it is heavenly - my body is smiling and I feel I do not need to breathe (until this point my breath has been heavy)
No time, no thoughts, no emotions. Bliss.

At one point, it strikes me that ordinarily in great happiness, tears come - why do they come? Perhaps in knowing it will end, or in sorrow at how things have not been this way all along? Anyway, in this state there are no tears.

Beyond emotion.
Pure consciousness.
I feel my question 'Who am I?' is being answered here - as much as I am currently able to know it.

Gethyn asks if I want another journey, I request a little more time. I am aware of where I am but able to remain in the bliss.

Second Run:
I ask if we can try to go deeper.
During the blissful state there was no imagery.
Now, I am back in a spirit realm - I feel angels around me - golden - thousands - a vast space - the angels are beneath and behind me. I am confronting the edge of God.

*I am being lifted up - my eyes are rolled back in my head - it feels further than I would be able to roll them back myself. (Later Gethyn reminds me of a story about a prisoner who believed that because when you die your eyes roll back, if he could roll his own back, he would see what the dead see - he practiced daily - then one night they rolled further than before and he had a spiritual experience and vision!)**

My body feels as if it is literally lifting off the couch - losing weight - I think if the couch had been a weighing scales, you would have seen the weight decrease. I feel like I could levitate. In the spirit realm I am moving slowly, very slowly, closer to God. It has to be this way so I can adjust - like slowly putting a hand in hot water so your body adjusts to the heat.

I feel humble yet worthy because I feel my true self is being given this. I feel clear.

Slowly now, I feel the experience is coming to an end, simply because I need to return.
I gently lower my body to the [massage] couch.
I return - ecstatic!
And revitalized.
And with the knowledge that this was more than a lucid dream - a real, true experience.
Wow."

* This story is from the book "Love Can Open Prison Doors" by Starr Daily, who, while in prison, sat with a dying man who had a spiritual experience as he died and his eyes rolled upward. Starr Daily then practised this after reading that "when the eyeballs were lifted upward in meditation we entered into the superconscious realm". With practice he claimed to be able to roll his eyes up to a single focal point in the centre of the forehead and have the same spiritual experience as the dying man.

What Do You Mean "Nothing Happened"?

Fortunately, the first clients to frame questions did get answers, ideas and inspiration. But when I eventually had clients who told me "nothing happened", there seemed to be several reasons why it 'didn't work'. Here I will address some common factors that inhibit the process.

The basic premise for Penetrating Heaven is that the answers are within us if only we can relax enough, in mind and body, and that Zero Balancing is a great way to relax deeply.

Relaxing the mind begins in framing the session, building a good Donkey connection, and addressing any concerns or potential obstacles on the path before the client even lies down.

Relaxing the body begins on the massage table. If nothing happens in the Intro Run, it can be because the client is not yet relaxed enough physically, and so they simply need more Zero Balancing to help them to relax and feel better in their own body.

So the client needs to be as comfortable and relaxed as possible. It may be something simple like putting a pillow under their knees, dimming the lights or offering them a blanket to help them to relax physically, but also to feel safe and secure, cocooned for their journey.

Many Shamanic journey practices begin with closing your eyes and taking a deep breath. Rona began her session with quick shallow breathing and later admitted she had felt anxious at first. So this is something to watch for. If I notice that the client is holding their breath or breathing shallowly at the beginning of the session, just before the Intro Run, then I will suggest that they take a nice deep breath. Usually the HMV at the feet and neck will have elicited a big breath before I start the Intro Run anyway but it is always good to observe the client for signs of discomfort, anxiety or nervousness that could inhibit them.

Of course, relaxing the mind and body go together, and Zero Balancing is ideal for both.

Mental tension from a busy brain, nervous expectation, mental chatter, being unable to switch off, over-thinking or trying too hard - these are all obstacles that tend to resolve with more time on the table, and more Zero Balancing, as the client relaxes and lets go.

Sometimes a client may have a physical issue that makes it difficult for them to relax and this may inhibit the process. So I also try to address any pain or physical tension first, especially in the neck, because I found that if I attempted a Run but nothing happened, then neck tension often seemed to be present. And this often coincided with mental tension, too.

If the client feels that nothing is happening, then usually they just need more Zero Balancing and more time before attempting another Run. It gets easier as the session progresses.

Occasionally one or two of my regular clients had a session where "not much happened" despite good previous sessions, and this coincided with them being over-tired or run down. In such cases, the body seems to prioritise what it needs and uses the session as an opportunity for rest, sleep and healing rather than going off on a journey somewhere.

So it really depends on how the client is and where they are at. What usually happens is that they get what they need, and what they are capable of handling on the day.

The Neck

(A Bridge Between Heaven and Earth)

From my observations and client feedback, the neck seems to be important in accessing altered states of consciousness, and in whether or not anything happens with Penetrating Heaven.

Back when I started using the Intro Run and weaving it into the Protocol, I gave a session to my friend Claire. I sat down behind her and launched straight into Penetrating Heaven. Although she had had plenty of sessions before (and did not have any neck restriction), she got very little response and remarked "You usually do more work on my neck first", suggesting to me that I should at least do the neck evaluations. This was good advice!

In Acupuncture most of the Window of Heaven points are located in the neck area, which is considered to be the 'bridge' between the head (Heaven) and the rest of the body (Earth). Energy can get stuck here, so it makes sense to release neck tension first in order to ensure that the energy is flowing more freely and that there is good communication between the head and the body, through the terrain of the Window of Heaven points.

Even when someone does not have any discernible neck tension or restriction, working on the neck is still useful because it can help to relax the person generally and it builds trust and a good Donkey connection, and this facilitates the Penetrating Heaven experience.

As I offered Penetrating Heaven to more people, I noticed that it sometimes didn't work so well if the client was holding a lot of tension in their neck, especially if they were also anxious by nature, wanting to stay in control, holding on, and being mostly 'up in their head'.

In such cases I would do more Zero Balancing for the neck, and I found that the "Baby OA" fulcrum that I had learned in the Secrets of the Skull workshop was especially useful for this. The Baby OA refers to the occiput and the atlas (the first vertebra of the neck). This fulcrum is a gentle hold, with one hand cradling the occiput and the fingers of the other hand placed on the vertebrae of the neck. In this way you stay at the Blue Line and meet any tension there, and by placing your awareness in your hands in this position, it allows the neck to balance itself.

(See also: "Zero Balancing Expanded: The Attitude of Awaiting a Fish" by Judith Sullivan)

I also remembered Fritz saying that neck problems will often respond if you put in a good rib fulcrum in the upper back, and I found that for some clients "nothing happened" until I had done so.

People with neck tension or restriction can still access altered state experiences, and still get answers! But the process does seem to improve greatly with a little more attention to the neck area.

During my ZB certification one of my case studies had a stiff neck, presenting with only about 10 degrees rotation left and right. By the end of the session, it had increased to a mere 20 degrees. I was quite disappointed until my mentor, Tim, pointed out that her neck rotation had doubled! And her own experience was much greater freedom and movement. Her feedback was that she "felt like an owl!" So the state of the neck is relative to the client and what they consider to be their own personal 'normal'. It can depend on the person's relationship with their neck, and perhaps whether their neck tension is of mental/emotional origin or of a physical origin.

Perhaps the sensation of more freedom, no matter how 'small', gives the person the space in which they can receive answers. It opens up that space for something new to come in.

Further Facilitating Fulcrums

If the client is mostly 'up in their head', with a busy brain that keeps them on a mental level rather than in their physical body, and if they "can't switch off", then I may use some of the Brain Fulcrums. Floating the Brain or Two Become One seem to work best for this.

Floating the Brain is a gentle supportive hold, with one hand cradling the occiput while the other hand on the frontal bone (forehead) is engaged in gentle compression, with the focus on the brain floating in the matrix of fascia and cerebral-spinal fluid within the skull.

Two Become One is a fulcrum with one hand at Bregma and the other hand at Lambda. Bregma is the meeting of the coronal and sagittal sutures on the midline of the skull. Lambda is the meeting of the lambdoid and sagittal sutures on the midline of the skull. These two locations can be gently held using the thumb of each hand.

(See also: "Zero Balancing Expanded: The Attitude of Awaiting a Fish" by Judith Sullivan)

If you are using the Baby OA, then you already have one hand under the occiput of the head and you can easily follow on into Floating the Brain, which gives the client a feeling of being held and being safe to let go. It is very relaxing, so it can be good to do before doing Penetrating Heaven. If you do it afterwards, the effect seems to be more containing rather than expansive.

When I experimented with Brain Fulcrums, I discovered that, while doing Two Become One - with my thumbs on Bregma and Lambda - my fingers could naturally fall into position for Tian Chong, GB-9 (as well as Shuaigu, GB-8). So this became a combination that I would sometimes use if nothing was happening, or if I thought the client was anxious, with a busy brain, worrying about their frame, or trying too hard.

So, for the Intro Run I would do Two Become One combined with Tian Chong, GB-9 (and also Shuaigu, GB-8), and then after a while I would take my thumbs away from Bregma and Lambda, and finally detach from Shuaigu, GB-8, in order to focus my middle fingers solely on Tian Chong, GB-9.

Early in my experimental sessions I had explored the use of Yin Tang, the Third Eye point, which I then abandoned in favour of Tian Chong, GB-9. However, during the development of Penetrating Heaven I was having regular sessions of Ayurvedic Yoga Massage, which included massaging in small circles along the Governing Vessel (the midline of the head), starting from the crown and slowly working towards massaging my Third Eye. This always had a powerful effect on me, sending me into a dream-like altered state of consciousness. So sometimes during Penetrating Heaven, if not much happens after a Run, I may follow up with massaging the Third Eye. This often stimulates visual images or makes the client's experience more visual, if it wasn't already. Some clients who saw fleeting images found that my finger on their Third Eye held the images stable, giving them more focus. When I removed my finger the images would disperse.

While researching Penetrating Heaven I came across the book "Windows of the Mind" by Gerald Glaskin, which describes the Christos Method of mind travel. This simple, effective technique involves massaging the ankles and Third Eye area simultaneously (with the help of an assistant). It reminded me of what Fritz Smith told us previously about two apparently opposing stimuli applied at the same time leading to an expanded state of consciousness. (See page 7-8)

I have used the Christos Method successfully without an assistant by simply doing a mini Zero Balancing session (about 10 minutes) and then massaging the client's Third Eye before continuing with the rest of the Christos Method, which guides the client through some simple visualization exercises. This can produce some fascinating and memorable journey experiences.

Facilitating Fields

Earlier, on page 74, I mentioned the Parallel Breath Meditation that Fritz teaches. I practise this for myself at home and also in my clinic to help me to stay clear, aligned and focused during my working day.

Later I began to use Parallel Breaths in Penetrating Heaven sessions to help me to stay focused and hold the space during a Run. And in time, I started to use it as one of my gears to introduce a clearer, stronger field as I touch the points.

Fritz also teaches how to breathe parallel breaths through a problem or situation. To do this, you first imagine placing the issue in your energy centre, or lower Dan Tien. Visualizing the problem there, you then begin to breathe parallel breaths through it. If you don't want the issue to be in your energy field, then you can place it out in front of your Dan Tien instead.

One day during a session, while I sat at the client's head, it occurred to me that my client happened to be right in front of my lower Dan Tien. Zero Balancing acts on the client's field - by putting in a clearer, stronger field - and the question (and answer) are in the client's field. So what would happen if I were to breathe parallel breaths through my client's framed question or issue?

This client wanted clarity on her relationship with her boyfriend, which she thought was about to end. She had lots of questions about how Penetrating Heaven works and said: "I'm no good at this." After a few Runs she said she didn't get anything, "just thoughts", and it didn't look as though she was going to get her answer. But then I had the idea to try something that I had not thought of before - to do the Parallel Breath meditation 'for her'.

I tried one more Run of Penetrating Heaven and took my hands away. Then I started breathing parallel breaths through her situation, in her field (in front of my lower Dan Tien as I sat behind her head).

As I did so, I noticed a small tear forming in the corner of her right eye. I continued to breathe parallel breaths through her issue, not touching her. Slowly this tear welled up and grew until finally the dam burst and she had a breakthrough! She saw images of friends and felt a sense of care, that she is cared for by friends, but also the question of whether her boyfriend cares.

"That sense of either my boyfriend caring - or that I need him to care - was strong."

And then she had a memory of a holiday trip with her boyfriend where she wanted to visit a tourist site but he didn't want to go, so she had gone with a "random guy" who was also on the same tour. While there, she had a photo taken with this guy and in this photo "We look like a couple but aren't!" As she said these words out loud, she realized that she had just described her current situation with her boyfriend, "We look like the perfect couple but the feeling isn't there."

A few days after this session her relationship ended, but the insight and clarity she received helped her to realize that it was for the best. She had gone into the session with a question and received her answer, and then applied it to her life.

Sometimes, if Penetrating Heaven still 'doesn't work', then perhaps the client needs help in 'forging a channel'. This will be discussed next.

Forging a Channel

Earlier, I discussed a few common themes that can occur in Penetrating Heaven, including childhood memories which John Lockley said can reveal our natural tendencies and gifts. Sarah's first session (below) was an example of such an experience. She said it reminded her of who she really was - before she grew up and learned to cover up her true self.

She reconnected with how she was as a young girl - expressive, always singing, dancing and entertaining people, which was later repressed because it annoyed her siblings, but this was the real her. Afterwards she felt like she had just had surgery, "split open, visible and seen".

Sarah said that each time we did a Run of Penetrating Heaven it became easier for her to access this altered state of consciousness, and it seemed to reinforce the effect. Each Run seems to make the subsequent Runs easier. She described this as "forging a channel" to the place of her experience.

Sarah (Session 1)

"The big question for me, for a very long time, has been:
'What should I be doing with my life?'
How hard can that be to answer?

I also have been scuppered by my Father's death, and the aftermath and backlash of family, and responsibilities coming out of my ears! Amazingly, my friends and children have been the kindest, whilst my siblings the harshest.

So, this Zero Balancing and Punching a Hole up to Heaven have been both timely and very welcome… Thank you!

I found it hard to let go and allow myself to get into the whole thing. But I know that every time you took me back in, I was forging a channel to somewhere much better than I've been, and certainly it connected me to my childhood happiness and the joy and power that came with that time in my life. I was able to look beyond the fear and the oppression that I feel in my family group, and reconnect with ME!

I was totally in my body (in my mind, ironically) and could feel myself dancing, singing and getting into physical action, being myself.

I also found myself being encouraged to be brave and bold, and to have opinions that I wanted to share, to end the silence that I enforce on myself. I felt freedom and that I could 'BE Happiness'. Also, it led me into believing that I am worthy and that I can ask for, or even demand, something for myself and that that would not be unreasonable. Also, that very notion of pleasing myself, which I have always steeped in guilt, melted away.

It also made me know that I would like to spend time with quieter people, so that I can be heard - something that I have not been able to do in a very long time.

In short, I am thinking about ways to bring all of this to life, every day; and I think that meditation would be very good for me, and the pursuit of joy.

*At the end of the session, it seemed that I had been laid out on a slab and opened up from throat to groin, which sounds dreadful, but it was actually the most wonderful feeling of freedom, since there could be no hiding what's inside me! Symbolically, it felt like I had just run naked through the streets telling everyone to 'F*ck off!' And it felt good!"*

Forging a Channel By Reinforcing a Run

Some clients, especially first-timers, can tend to go in and out of the altered state and may need a bit of help to take them back there. Therefore, I might sometimes do several short repeat Runs, one after the other, to reinforce the effect and help the person in this way.

After her first session Sarah told me that having several repeat Runs helped, and that it was good to "come out and go back in again". It became easier, like she was "forging a channel" to 'get there', to 'get to that place'. But she said that it was also her will to do so, she wanted to.

Another client, Laura, said she "dipped in and out of it" at first. She went deep but resisted and "came back again". Having a few short, repeated Runs, one after the other, helped her to 'practice' going there and get accustomed to it.

The Intro Run is, of course, just an introduction. It can help to gauge the client's response and to identify obstacles. It could also be used as an opportunity to experiment with forging a channel, with repeat Runs, but usually I don't worry if nothing much happens this early in the session.

In the later Runs, however, if it feels necessary (i.e. if the effect is fluctuating or fading), then I may repeat Penetrating Heaven and touch the points again to reinforce the Run, and to forge a channel. Several short repeat Runs one after the other can really help.

Forging a Channel With Several Runs Within a Session

Typically, most clients will go into an altered state and receive their answers at some stage, sometimes even as early as in the Intro Run. But generally their experience will get better, and go deeper, with each successive Run as the session progresses. This may be because of the accumulative effect of having had more Zero Balancing, which helps the client to relax more deeply as we go along. Also, the client has had more time to process what is happening.

Weaving several Runs into a session gives Penetrating Heaven an accumulative effect as well, as each Run builds on the previous Run(s). Through this, the client is able to forge a channel for accessing their experience. And the channel builds as I give the client more time for each Run. Each successive Run is longer, which allows the client more time to have their experience. And longer Runs tend to go deeper.

If the client is resisting or blocking the experience, then repeat Runs early in the session can reassure them that they are in control. They learn that there is nothing to worry about and so they relax into it. And, of course, they know they can have a few more goes later in the session.

From session feedback I know that, if the client is eager to have an experience and trying too hard, telling them that they can have more than one Run at it is helpful because it takes the pressure off the person "to have an experience". It is not a one chance deal, and so the client can have 'practice runs' to experiment and get used to the process, thereby building confidence.

Forging a Channel Over Several Sessions

Even though the first session can yield answers and amazing transformative experiences, most of my regular clients have told me that it is helpful to have more than one session. By forging a channel over a course of several sessions, the experience gets even better and clients say they are able to 'get there' quicker, and 'go deeper' the more sessions they have: "It gets easier to drop into that space." It's like establishing a path: The more often you walk the path and clear away obstacles along it, the easier the journey gets.

In Zero Balancing, and the Bowen Technique, the body seems to remember any work it has received in the past. And because it has had the experience before, it responds quicker in subsequent sessions. This is also true for Penetrating Heaven. Regular clients seem to drop into 'that space' a lot more quickly and easily, and earlier in the session. It is like practicing stretches in yoga: The more you do it, the further you can go, and it becomes quicker and easier each time.

Many of my regular clients tell me that sessions can follow on from each other, or that they can have a recurring theme, even if they are weeks, or months, apart.

Miranda felt her second session progressed further and built on her first: *"My second session seemed to follow on quite naturally from the first. I received greater clarity on some of the questions I'd posed in the first session in that some of the symbols were similar in nature but now richer in detail. Some of them morphed into other symbols and seemed to show me how things might develop over time, despite how they might initially appear on the surface."*

Barbara also felt that her second session picked up where her first session had left off. Both of her sessions shared a similar theme, but she told me that this was not something she had thought about during the weeks in between the sessions. She believed that Penetrating Heaven had given her something that she didn't normally have access to.

Forging a Channel With Client's Donkey

Forging a channel can also be a case of building trust and a good Donkey Connection, with the client becoming more familiar with how sessions work, and letting go and trusting the process.

After a Run or two, or a session or two, the client grows more used to the altered states. They feel less anxious and drop their inhibitions, and as a result they find it is easier to let go and surrender into the experience. They can go deeper and explore further, being more willing and enthusiastic to journey.

The Zero Balancing Protocol follows the same regular routine sequence in every session, so it can quickly become familiar to the client. This helps their Donkey to feel safe and reassured. A familiar ritual can elicit the same feelings we have had before when it is repeated, and it can make us anticipate a similar experience to the one that occurred in the past. This is why some athletes will repeat ritual routines to 'psyche themselves up' while preparing for an event.

NLP (Neuro-Linguistic Programming) shows that people can be conditioned to associate certain stimuli (visual, kinaesthetic or auditory) with a certain feeling by simple repetition. For example: If, each time you feel happy, you make a certain facial expression, feel a certain touch or hear a certain sound (or catchphrase), then eventually you will associate them with each other, and that stimuli can then be used to elicit the same happy feeling. This is called an Anchor.

The same principle works in Penetrating Heaven. The client builds an association with the expanded states of consciousness through the Anchors that I set by the fact that Penetrating Heaven is woven into the regular Zero Balancing Protocol routine, with my 'ritual' of touching the point, Tian Chong, GB-9, in the same way each time, and with my habit of using the same phrases to talk to the client. When a regular client returns for a session, these Anchors set the scene for a repeat.

Regular clients also get to know me, and become more familiar with the venue, as well as the whole process and how it feels, so they are more relaxed to begin with. They know what to expect, and because of this they trust the process more, relaxing into it quicker, and letting go.

So, for experienced regular clients who have had Penetrating Heaven before, and who have already forged a channel in previous sessions, it gets easier to go deeper each time, and to access these expanded states of consciousness more quickly, and earlier in the session - sometimes from just the Introductory Run, after minimal Zero Balancing (although exactly how much Zero Balancing the client needs will depend on where they are at on the day).

Some seasoned regular clients who have had lots of sessions with me in the past seem to go into an expanded state of consciousness almost immediately and at the slightest touch of the points, before I even feel I've got into gear! In such cases I use a lighter touch and take my hands away sooner because otherwise I can inhibit the experience as the client is taking off.

So, the Penetrating Heaven effect seems to get better the more sessions a person has, partly because of the repeated practice in 'forging a channel'. Another possible reason why the experiences grow ever deeper is that, as obstacles fall away, my regular clients start to expand on what they ask for in their framed questions, inviting more profound experiences.

At first they start small with their questions, but in later sessions they push beyond their limitations and expand their horizons, asking: "What else is possible?" Or they may ask some of the bigger fundamental questions of life. Perhaps the only limitations are the ones we place on ourselves, so we get the experience that we allow ourselves to have.

The Client and the Practitioner

As I did more sessions with people, I noticed some parallels between my client and myself, i.e. what was happening for the client, and what was happening with me.

Earlier I mentioned obstacles on the path - reasons why the client may impede the process - but sometimes I needed to acknowledge the obstacle in myself.

I want my client to relax, let go and trust the process. But I need to relax and trust myself, trust Zero Balancing and trust Penetrating Heaven. If I can do that then it serves my client.

I want my client to get out of their own way mentally, and let go of their stuff. But I had to learn to do this, too, and allow myself to be guided by the session, which sometimes meant breaking with the Protocol or trying something new. This was my own journey.

I want my client to be open to the answer coming in whatever form it appears, and the variety in their different experiences taught me to let go of how I think it is supposed to be.

I want my client to let go of their attachment to the outcome, but I needed to learn this, too. If I worry about 'results' or what 'should' happen, then I am not fully present in the moment. This was the hardest thing for me to accept because naturally I wanted my technique to work and be successful. In the beginning I took it very seriously, and I worried when it seemed that it wasn't working. Sometimes I wondered if anything was happening at all, and I earnestly tried hard to get a result. It was a relief when a client got an answer and gave me positive feedback after a Run because then I could relax - and it would be a better session. But I had to learn to let go of all of that inner tension. Ultimately the client's experience is not my responsibility.

My job is to provide a safe space and to hold the field in order to facilitate the client's experience. But I am aware of the parallels that can exist between myself and my client and the obstacles we both share - and it is my responsibility to deal with the obstacles in myself.

Of course, the parallels between my client and myself can also be positive and affirming:

Sometimes a client shares their answer with me, and it seems to apply to me, too. For example, a client received her answer "Let it go", which resonated with my own situation at the time. Another client said their answer was "Love", more specifically "Self-Love", which, again, on that day was particularly relevant to me.

I am trying to help facilitate the client in receiving insights and answers but often, within the setting of a session, in that container, it seems that I can go into an altered meditative state as well, and I will sometimes receive a stream of creative ideas of my own.

Zero Balancing and Penetrating Heaven open people up so that they can access parts of themselves they may not ordinarily be aware of. But practising it on others has opened me up, too. How could it be any different?

The different stages of a session can also contain parallels between the client and myself:

The whole ritual routine serves as a familiar Anchor to help the client in the process, and it also helps me. My way of finding the points and arranging my fingers helps to put me into the right state of mind, as well.

The Intro Run serves as a warm-up or practise run for the client, and it is also there to help iron out any obstacles for the person early on. But it serves as all of these things for me, too.

Just as the client forges a channel, sometimes it feels that I am forging a channel, too. With each Run and each session I am becoming more practiced, getting into my groove.

Holding Space

One day I was giving my friend Iren a session at her house. Conditions were not ideal as there were several distractions. She had just put the washing outside to dry, and as the session began we heard it starting to rain heavily. Meanwhile her dogs, Ralph and Rocky, wanted to be in on the session, too. They were growling, playing and wanting attention, occasionally bumping into the table legs as I sat, ever so seriously, working on Iren.

From less than perfect situations comes perfect learning. Iren said that she could feel it when I got distracted or annoyed by the dogs. She said she had felt my attention waver and the effect had faded. This made me appreciate even more how important my field is, i.e. my attention - it is not just about touch with attention, but I must hold the space with attention, too.

I know from receiving massages and other bodywork that you can often sense if the practitioner hesitates, or if something breaks their concentration or interrupts their flow. The client knows!

In the early days of Penetrating Heaven, I would take my hands away to allow the Run and then spend those few minutes waiting and wondering if anything was happening, but once I knew that my technique worked, I resolved to use this time to maintain my own field and to hold the space with my attention. To be fully in the present moment is key to this!

The key to conscious touch is attention. Likewise, the key to holding space is attention. To hold the space during a Run means to adopt the role of sentinel: I look with “soft eyes” and pay attention. I observe the client and watch for working signs.

But there is a deeper aspect: I also pay attention to the unseen, feeling the ‘energy’ of the room. So I ask myself how the client is doing, and get a sense of whether anything is happening; or I ask myself if the client needs more time, and intuitively feel the subtle level of activity. I also stay alert and ready for any emotional release that may occur because this can sometimes happen, too.

Zero Balancing is a working meditation, and holding space can be a meditation as well. In order to help me hold the space and be in the present moment, I do the Parallel Breath Meditation.

Another technique is to imagine drawing a circle around the client and massage table, with the intention that it contains the person in a sacred space of privacy and protection where I cannot enter, interrupt or intrude. Drawing the circle reminds me to get out of the way! Initially I chose a circle because of some other energy work I had done but later I remembered that in Chinese Philosophy a circle represents Heaven.

As my work took me into more shamanic territory, I met practitioners who agreed with the need for focused attention so that you "don't lose the client". They also acknowledged the importance of taking steps for protection before a client journeys, such as the circle boundary I imagined, although I did this more for holding space and an intention of privacy rather than a perceived need for protection.

Sometimes, in my own meditative state, this circle seems to take on a life of its own and spirals into the shape of a cone or tipi, or it adopts a pyramid shape, pointing up to Heaven. This reinforces the idea of forging a channel to our higher consciousness as well as holding a particular space for the client.

In Zero Balancing we may start a group meeting or workshop with a pyramid meditation, visualizing a pyramid over the space we are in. The geometric form of the pyramid acts as a container to hold, focus and amplify our collective energy, thoughts and intention.

"Holding Space" means you are allowing the session to hold your attention, focus and awareness; it means listening, watching and sensing, and being ready to respond to your client, while remaining rooted in your own body.

In the Bowen Technique, the practitioner performs moves on the client's body and then waits for at least 2 minutes for them to process the work. During this time the practitioner may step outside of the room - they will certainly step outside of the client's space - to allow the process to work. But they always maintain their connection, and attention, to the client. So here, too, this quality of holding space is key.

Ralph and Rocky aside, most of my sessions take place in a quiet treatment room. However, sometimes I have done sessions in noisy environments, such as at festivals with music and general outside noise, or in a city centre clinic while buskers sang in the street below. On one occasion we had a local celebrity switching on the Christmas lights to cheering and applause. Usually any outside noise is more natural such as seagulls calling, the wind blowing, a dog barking or the rain falling.

If there is a lot of noise or distraction, either outside the room or within the client's mind, then I may hold their head or do a gently holding brain fulcrum like Floating the Brain or Two Become One. This will help to quieten the person, whether the noise is external or internal.

But it is not really the noise that is important. What is important is our relationship to it. For me as the practitioner, far from being a distraction, lots of noise or activity outside the room can serve to focus my attention even more. And it makes me more determined to reinforce the field and hold the space with attention.

As those who practice meditation will know, noise, distraction or discomfort are unavoidable at times. But these things are not to be resisted or rejected. Rather, we can acknowledge that they are there, accept them, and make them part of the meditation. We don't have to do anything about them but we can choose where we place our focus.

Sometimes I feared that the outside noise might spoil a client's experience, only to be told that it made perfect sense to them, and the outer activity reflected the client's inner experience. The sound of an accelerating motorbike, a police siren, a busker's song, or a crying child have been synchronistic and meaningful to the client, and very relevant to their question.

During one session, my client heard someone in the nearby nursery playground singing: "Get ready, get ready!" She told me that this tied in perfectly with her question. Another client, pondering his future at a workplace he didn't enjoy, heard a man's voice outside the window shouting: "Leave! Leave!" It was a passer-by issuing a command to his dog, but it had an obvious and timely significance to my client's answer.

Once the client sets a clear intention or question and put it into their Frame, the whole session and what happens in it seems to relate to the Frame and will resonate in some way. The Frame gives the client's experience a context.

When I have offered Zero Balancing and Penetrating Heaven at festivals, I have found myself working next to sound healers or gong baths, or my sessions have been accompanied by nearby drumming or the sound of didgeridoos. Instead of it being a distraction, my clients told me that these sounds became part of their inner journey and made their experience even more powerful.

Holding space was something I had already been doing naturally but now I acknowledged it as essential to the work and consciously made it part of my technique. And I used my attention to hold the space.

I see Holding Space as an extension of Hold, Listen, Allow: I hold my attention by being actively aware of what is occurring in the space; I 'listen' or sense for activity or changes, including working signs, and I allow whatever is happening to happen while holding it in my awareness.

Highest Personal Regard

Fritz teaches to hold each person, including yourself, "in the Highest Personal Regard". This means holding everyone with respect and high esteem, without judgement or comparison. (This idea will also be familiar to students of the psychologist Carl Rogers.)

The word "regard" comes from the French verb "regarder", which means "to look at" or "to watch". I had experimented with Highest Personal Regard by "holding" people with my eyes, without an agenda, without judgement, without imposition, by simply allowing them to be as they are. I find it very powerful to be a sentinel, holding space with my eyes. Once, after a workshop at Gaunts, I observed two strangers arguing in a café. I held them in the Highest Personal Regard and witnessed a dramatic transformation take place as peace quickly descended on their table. Coincidence?

"When you change the way you look at things,
the things you look at change."
- Max Planck

Obviously in bodywork we can hold a person physically, for example hold their rib cage or hold their feet or head, and do so with the Highest Personal Regard. We can also hold a person in the Highest Personal Regard mentally, in our thoughts and our attitude towards them.

And we can also hold a person with our gaze, which can be seen as a form of touch, too. According to my school science teacher, when we look at someone we see them because tiny particles of light called photons are bouncing off them and into our eyes, touching the retina in our eye to produce an image in our brain. So when you truly look at a person, without judgement or agenda, holding them in the Highest Personal Regard, then you are already touching, at least on a microscopic quantum level.

So the first touch is with the eyes. There is contact and interface.

Most people will have had the experience of knowing when somebody is watching them. And they will somehow know exactly where that person is, and turn to look straight at them. This phenomenon is explored in "The Sense of Being Stared At" by Rupert Sheldrake. I have been told that Special Forces soldiers, in escape and evade training, are instructed not to look directly at their pursuer when hiding. We *feel* it when someone is looking at us.

When I learned a little Shiatsu, I was taught about the idea of sending one's Ki (energy) through a client's body by one's eyes and intention. We can affect another person with our eyes.

Fritz advises us to "look with soft eyes", allowing the image of the person to enter our eyes rather than actively looking. In contrast, I have heard border collie sheepdogs described as having a 'hard eye' (or 'strong eye'), enabling them to move stubborn sheep with a penetrating stare and an attitude. (Some dogs are even said to have 'too much eye'!) Staring is aggressive and intrusive, not healing, so we soften our focus.

So we can Hold Space with our eyes...
This is what led me to visualizing a circle of protection around my clients - to hold them and allow them to have their experience, while I act as sentinel and watch for working signs.

... and we can hold the other person in the Highest Personal Regard with our eyes.
Hold Space with your eyes but also hold the person in the Highest Personal Regard. This is easier to do if you look at their face. Connect with them as a person, feel compassion and respect for them, so you are fully engaged and attentive. Bring Highest Personal Regard into your gaze.

What I Learned from Animals

The following encounter illustrates the importance of these ideas of holding space and connection with the eyes and our attention:

One morning I was sitting on Hove beach when I met a woman walking her two boxer dogs, an old, slow one and a young, playful one. The young one came over to say hello to me but then quickly ran off to explore the beach. The older one still lagged behind. I chatted to the woman for a while as the old boxer finally caught up and came over to say hello to me, shoving her face affectionately into mine before she continued on her way towards the woman who was still facing me, talking. The dog was between me and the woman and turned back to face me, with her back to the woman, who said goodbye to me and turned away to continue her walk. At the very moment the woman turned her back on me, the dog suddenly started barking at me, warning me off as I sat there quietly on the beach. She had sensed the disconnect. The woman was no longer engaged with me - it was like flicking a switch. The woman turned back to see what was wrong and took control of the situation, so all was well again. But it showed that the dog had sensed that the space between the owner and me was no longer held.

In my own experience of receiving bodywork - Zero Balancing and massage - I know that when lying down relaxed with my eyes closed, I can sense if the practitioner hesitates or interrupts their flow, and there is an unseen disturbance in the session.

Sometimes I have given sessions in a room where the clock is behind me so I have had to turn around, with my back to the client, to check the time. This temporarily breaks the link and the client may feel it affect their experience so this is something to be mindful of.

.....

The Trusting Donkey and the Intuitive Horse

One year after Richard had facilitated my first journey, I was still working on my Penetrating Heaven technique and still trying to find my way along my dark muddy path. My clinic was going well - but something was amiss and I couldn't quite put my finger on it. I had a new client who couldn't run because he was in pain, which meant he had to give up playing sports and his social life around that. I gave him Acupuncture and the next day he ran to catch a train. He was delighted. And I should have been, too. All through my training I had dreamt of helping people like this. But despite getting the results, I wasn't happy in my heart. So, I decided to try a session of equine therapy at Intuitive Horse on a farm near Hastings. (It was 2014, the year of the Horse, which relates to the heart in Chinese Philosophy!)

Horses are prey animals, so they need to be constantly alert and attuned to their environment as well as to those in their company. In other words, they have to be present in the moment. And in order to interact with horses successfully, we have to be in the present moment as well. These animals are very sensitive and can 'read' people; they have the ability to detect the slightest tension in humans. And they mirror our mental-emotional state back to us, which makes them good therapists!

Emma, the equine therapy facilitator, began our session with a discussion about my reasons for coming. We talked about my vague dissatisfaction and frustration, and the disconnect or lack of fulfilment that I felt. I was not enjoying success; there was an incongruence, and that became my 'Frame'.

Next we stood in the farmyard, and Emma guided me through a meditative body scan. Standing comfortably, I was led to focus my attention on different parts of my body in turn, head to toes, until I noticed where I felt a sensation. I felt something, a block, a heaviness, a ball of 'something', in my sternum in the centre of my chest. This became my marker, something in my physical body for me to monitor and receive feedback from; I was to keep noticing if it changed during the session.

Then we went over to the herd to choose a horse for me to work with. I stood with my back to them, checked in with the feeling in my sternum, then turned around to see if I was drawn to a particular horse. The feeling in my sternum intensified when I looked at Harvey, a magnificent grey, and it faded when I looked away. So I chose Harvey. (Or had he chosen me?)

Emma led Harvey out from the herd into an enclosed, walled yard. And I was invited to interact with him. He didn't seem very keen and stood with his back to me at the exit gate.

It began as a tense stand-off. I was nervous, unsure what to do. I walked towards Harvey and tried all sorts of strategies to make friends with him, talking softly, varying my distance from him, trying to position myself so he would have to connect with me. Nothing worked. He stood with his back to me, facing the exit gate, and just seemed intent on getting back to his herd. I felt rejected. But I did notice the ball in my sternum starting to soften... And I recognised it as sadness - sadness for my situation, grieving because it was different to how I thought it would be.

I gave up. I walked back to Emma who was sitting in the shade in the corner, out of the way. She asked me how it was going. I just shrugged: "He doesn't want to play with me." In that moment I dropped all of my strategising and my whole agenda... and immediately I heard hoof steps behind me and Harvey's nose appeared on my shoulder.

What had just happened? I had given up, let go, dropped all of my agenda, expectations and tension. And I had acknowledged and expressed how I was feeling, yes feeling, in the present moment - and instantly Harvey had turned and trotted over to me.

I stroked Harvey, he nudged me back, then nuzzled me. It was so powerful and overwhelming, there was a sense of real meaningful affection - it was very emotional. As I was analysing what had happened, Harvey went away and rolled on his back in the sand as if to say: "Loosen up! Enjoy it!"

Once I had acknowledged this, he came again and stamped his hoof emphatically at me, which I took to mean: "Come on! That's it, you've got it! Life is that simple. Now come on!" I had not been appreciating what I had; I was not celebrating how far I had come.

I felt relief at this breakthrough. Harvey nuzzled me again and I felt happy, and I noticed that what was left of that blocked feeling in my sternum had dissolved and cleared completely.

Harvey only really interacted and engaged with me when I was present in the moment, or when I forgot myself and got lost in the moment, rather than planning or strategising future goals.

When I surrendered and stopped trying so hard, when I just dropped my baggage and let go, Harvey sensed it and responded.

The session was liberating, and I left the farm feeling happier than I had been for a long time.

Some time later I did a home visit for an Acupuncture client. On arriving at the house, her dog, Pancake, greeted me excitedly and then lay down quietly on her bed by the fire, watching me work. I was busy up in my head working out my diagnosis and selecting which Acupuncture points to use but once I had decided on the points and needled them, there was a moment when I dropped all that mental stuff and went into free flow. Pancake instantly sensed this and ran over to me again for some attention.

What I learned from these experiences with animals helped to explain and confirm something that I was beginning to notice: The best sessions of Penetrating Heaven are the ones in which I am able to relax, drop my stuff and let go. I need to get out of the way - and that includes letting go of the outcome or the result.

The Field of the Practitioner

The session with Harvey felt like the best treatment I had ever received. I went home feeling like something in me had changed, and the ripple effect continued for a long time afterwards. I also went away thinking that Harvey must be just about the best therapist in the world! But what makes him so good? He didn't really do anything... Or did he?

No, Harvey didn't do anything. He was simply being. He was being himself, his true nature, authentic. His was a clearer, stronger field, and his attention was in the present moment.

In order to interact with him I had to drop my stuff, i.e. my thoughts of the past or future, and be in the present moment with him. Only then could we start to build a relationship.

A Cranio-Sacral Therapist once told me: "We heal in relationship to." Life is about relationships - our relationship with our self, our environment, and whoever we share this moment with.

The way Harvey relates to the world is authentic. He is clear about who he is, and this acted as a mirror for me. Harvey didn't want anything from me. He didn't have an agenda, he didn't want the session to go a particular way, and he wasn't trying to achieve anything. He wasn't attached to the 'result' of the session and he didn't take on any responsibility for it. He was free of all of this. Therefore, he could be fully present in the moment, and he left it up to me to choose whether I met him there or not. Everything happens in the present moment.

In Quantum Touch, the practitioner uses the breath to raise their energetic state to a higher vibration than that of the client, who may then adopt this higher vibration by 'Entrainment'. Entrainment, as explained earlier, works in a similar way to when a note is played on a piano and a guitar placed nearby will sound the same note by resonance. This same phenomenon can also be demonstrated by using two tuning forks.

We affect each other, it is just a question of who holds their vibrational field the steadiest. And if you as the practitioner can consistently stay in a higher vibration for long enough, then the client will 'give up'! Some practitioners are like chameleons and adapt to their client, which is one way of working; other practitioners are like a rock, constant and uncompromising, so that their client's 'wave' breaks on that rock.

My breakthrough at Intuitive Horse happened when I gave up, let go and dropped my stuff. Harvey's stance, his clear field, helped me to do that, not by force but by sheer gentle, irrepressible strength.

In Zero Balancing a fulcrum introduces a clearer, stronger vibrational field with unwavering constancy, and around this still point the client's energy has the opportunity to re-organize itself. The constancy is achieved by the practitioner being authentic, congruent and true.

Clearer, stronger fields can provide us with opportunities for healing and transformation. Harvey radiated a clearer, stronger field, and it was easy for him to maintain the constancy because he was simply being himself, expressing his true nature, in the present moment. He didn't need to drop anything. I did. And I gave up and let go. And I received the healing.

Harvey wasn't using any technique, he was simply being. Through him I saw that healing is not just about a technique but very much about the present moment, authenticity, and relationship. It is also about how much the practitioner is able to fully be their self, their true self, in what they do.

It is also about the heart. As I explained earlier, in Acupuncture the heart is seen as the Emperor, that part of Heaven in us whose role it is to be a void (i.e. open, clear and uncluttered), so that from this calm stillness our authentic sovereign self can shine through.

My experience with Harvey made me, as a practitioner, appreciate even more how important my own vibrational field is. Penetrating Heaven began with me connecting to the Stillness Field, holding it in myself and offering it to the client. And although I found different ways of doing this (my different gears), I realised that the key is not so much the technique I use but how much it helps me to be in my own field.

As described earlier, I had noticed parallels between myself and my client. There is not only the field of the practitioner and the field of the client, there is also the shared field of the session. It is in this shared field where these parallels occur, and if I can take care of my own field, it will support my client's experience. By being clear in myself, I enable the other person's journey by acting as a 'tuning fork' for them.

'Taking care of my own field' begins on a physical level, being mindful of my posture throughout the session, being aware of any tension I may hold in my body and consciously softening and relaxing my muscles. My breathing is also part of this process of relaxing and enhancing my own field, both as I do the Zero Balancing Protocol and as I consciously use my breath in applying my gears.

I am aware of my weight on the chair, feeling my feet on the floor, and rooting myself in my own body. Sometimes I imagine roots going down into the earth. After a session one of my clients said that she had seen me as a tree, rooted in the Earth, reaching up to Heaven.

On a mental level, I will pause to centre myself and silently acknowledge my own intention or frame for the session: that I do my job to the best of my ability, relaxed, open and present. My wish is that my client will receive what they need or let go of what they no longer need. I have already described holding space and imagining a circle of privacy and protection, and opening my heart to hold the client in the Highest Personal Regard with compassion.

So, in the analogy of the practitioner as a tree, I am reaching up to Heaven while remaining rooted in the Earth, casting a circle of protective shelter over my client while I hold space, reinforcing and maintaining the strength and clarity of my own field throughout the session.

Penetrating Heaven is built on the premise that the answers are within if we will only relax and get out of the way mentally, and if we let go, creating the space and the stillness that allow answers to arise. And if I, as the practitioner, am able to do this for myself, then it can help the client to do so, too.

My gears help me to do this. They help me to silence my monkey mind chatter and get out of the way mentally; to be in my feeling mind, not my thinking mind, creating space to be in stillness. It is a working meditation, keeping my mind in my fingertips at all times. And I am being present - attention in the present moment is a key element of Penetrating Heaven.

The gears that I have found to have the most powerful effect on the client are the ones that appeal to me personally - those that help me to fully engage and put me in touch with myself. Using my Heart Light puts my focus in my heart, that little bit of Heaven in me, the core of who I am, my authentic self; there is a field of stillness and clarity there. I have also found that a feeling of gratitude helps.

There are many ways of doing this kind of work but it's not really about the technique. What matters is how much you, the practitioner, are able to be yourself with the technique and express your true nature. In this way, you make the technique your own.

What Are You Doing When You Are Not Touching Me?

From the first experimental sessions with Penetrating Heaven, the feedback that I received was that I was ‘charging up’ the points and nothing happened until I took my hands away.

With a lighter touch the client can start to have an experience before I take my hands away. But it is in the pause, the 5-10 minutes that I allow for a Run, that the real magic happens.

And clients feel it. They ask me: “What are you doing when you are not touching me?”

My initial response was that I am not doing anything - I am only here to get out of the way! But this question felt important. There had to be more to it than that. Clients sense how powerful the pause is but they query it because the experience gets better when I am not touching them, so it must be coming from them!

“What were you doing when you took your hands off and just sat behind me? Because it was most powerful when your hands were off. That is when things really happened!”

When I take my hands away for a Run I am still holding the space, maintaining the field and watching for working signs. But I am not doing anything more for the client. I simply allow them the time and space to have their experience. And that’s the important part.

In Zero Balancing we don’t ‘do to’ the client but we ‘work with’ them. We are not trying to change anything and we are certainly not trying to force anything; instead we offer a fulcrum and allow things to unfold. We hold the fulcrum, listen with attention, and allow what happens to happen.

The Chinese term for this is Wu Wei (‘non action’). There is power in not ‘doing’ anything. It is not ‘doing nothing’ but it is not doing, i.e. not trying, not forcing, having no agenda and no attachment to a particular outcome. It is going with the nature of things.

When my dad taught me carpentry as a young boy, he watched me struggle as I tried to saw a piece of wood. He said "Let the saw do the work", and that made it much easier. Holding the saw loosely, not forcing or 'efforting' in any way, allowed the tool in my hand to do its job in a relaxed way.

And with Penetrating Heaven it is important to remember that I am not 'doing' or forcing anything. What I give in the session is an offering. In the early days, when I realized that my technique works, I began to relax and stopped trying so hard, i.e. I got out of the way! Today, I let go and give up control to the Stillness Field or my Heart Light, or whichever gear I am using. So, let the fulcrum do the work, and let the pause do the work.

Everything happens in the pause, when I am not doing any work but allowing the response to occur. The pause is as important as the work; a pause in the work allows a response in the Run.

A client once asked: "I don't understand. How can it work when you are not even touching me?" A garden still grows when you are not working in it. As a gardener, you do the work and plant the seeds and then it just needs time and a little tending. As a practitioner, I do the work and set things up and then give you time and a little guidance. There is no more to do.

Some of the best sessions are when I take my hands away and sit well back in my chair, with my hands in my lap, i.e. when I get out of the way (physically and mentally) and let go. I still hold the space but I relax and let the pause do the work, and I know and trust that the client is having their experience.

Questions for Exploring Symptoms

As more and more people received answers to their questions, and some even had the experience of journeying inside their body and seeing what was happening in their own anatomy, I wondered if Penetrating Heaven could be used to explore physical symptoms, to ask questions that might reveal the reasons for the client's health problems and to get more clarity on their condition. And perhaps to ask what the client may do as a next step toward health.

So I began to invite some clients to ask: "What do I need to know about my symptoms?"

Typical responses included images, symbols, memories of past events or old emotions which, when viewed from the perspective of the framed question, related to the client's symptoms.

I remembered that years ago I went to hear somebody speak about healing, and they said that an important part of healing is "letting go [of our dysfunctional habits or beliefs] and being prepared to see another way". Many people have had the experience of Zero Balancing giving them a new perspective, so I wondered if Tian Chong, GB-9, could help the client to look through another 'window' and see new possibilities for their health. And I remembered what Fritz had said about expanded states of consciousness helping us to let go:

> *"There are healing advantages of the expanded state because the person is less well held to their dysfunctions and therefore more able to change."*
>
> \- Dr Fritz Smith

So, a session can be used to frame a particular health issue and ask a question that is aimed at helping the client to see another way and get new insights into their health. Useful ways of phrasing the question are, for example:

"What do I need to know about my symptoms?" or "What is the cause of my symptoms?"

"What is going on with my health (or my body)?" or "What do I need to acknowledge?"

"What is stopping me from healing this?" or "What do I need to let go of in order to heal?"

If we can see what obstacles block our path to health, then we can ask what to do about it:

"What is my next step toward health?"

So, the client can explore if there is anything they need to know, or acknowledge, or let go of, or forgive.

Gaining an insight into our past experiences or our current situation can be therapeutic and transformational in itself, as we acknowledge our reality in the present moment. In some sessions the approach to touch - holding, listening and allowing - is beautifully reflected in how the client meets their condition: They hold it in their own mind, listen or feel into it, and just for a moment allow it to be as it is in the stillness of the session.

In this space, the client can invite a new perspective to emerge that will allow them to change their relationship to their situation. Through this, they may begin to see what else is possible and how things could perhaps be better.

Our Relationship With Our Symptoms

When clients explore the reasons for their symptoms and gain a new perspective on them, it can help them 'reset' or recalibrate their relationship to their condition.

For example, a client saw the reason for her migraines: "It is so that I stop, so that I am in the present moment, or so that I reconnect with nature, because that's what I do whenever I get one."

One client asked the question: "What do I need to know about my tinnitus?" And she received a new perspective on it, revealing: "My tinnitus is so that I don't get distracted." She explained that she felt able to use the condition to help her to focus, to harness it as a meditation.

Another client, also with tinnitus, said that after the session she felt more accepting of it, "not pushing it away", and "I was able to change my relationship to the tinnitus".

I had wondered, if a client is in pain, whether this might distract and prevent them from reaching that state where answers come from. But I need not have worried - they do still receive answers. Perhaps the response depends on the client's relationship to their pain and what they are used to. It is all relative.

Sometimes there is an emotional component to symptoms that needs to be acknowledged. Again, we ask what we can do about it, or if something from the past needs to be forgiven. Some examples follow.

.....

Sometimes the client may require a bit of help in exploring their symptoms, and I support their enquiry in the form of a dialogue:

A woman, aged 50, had a pain in her right hip, so she framed her question to ask: "What is the cause of my hip pain?" She immediately received the answer: "Fear. It's a fear paralysis." I asked: "Fear of what?"

And she replied: “Everything!” So I suggested asking “What’s the best thing to do about it?“ She saw the words “Let go” in the sky, but she did not know what to let go of. So I suggested that she ask what to let go of, and to ask for it in symbolic form.

She saw an image of an egg that was balancing upright with the sense that it was not safe to let go. I suggested that nature designed the egg to be such a shape that it won’t roll very far. But she didn’t want it to fall, so I suggested imagining it in an egg cup. But she didn’t want to rely on any external help. When I replied that it wouldn’t be external because it was coming from within her own sub-conscious mind, she imagined the egg stood upright in an egg cup, and it was now safe. After a few moments I asked how her hip was and she said that the pain was gone.

.....

As the above shows, the client can work with what comes up and use their imagination to envisage change. Here is another example of this:

A woman, aged 72, presented with pain and restriction in her right upper arm, so we framed the question for Penetrating Heaven as: “What do I need to know about my arm injury?” During the session the woman saw an image of an ash tree at the end of her garden, which was healthy except for one thin, withered branch. I encouraged her to imagine nourishing this branch so that it could grow strong and sprout leaves again, and as she visualized this, she told me the pain went away. I checked back some months later and she was still pain free.

Making Connections

My session with Harvey at Intuitive Horse began with me focusing on my problem and then doing a body scan in which I put my awareness in each part of my body in turn, from head to toe, to see if I could find any bodily representation of my issue. The purpose of this was to feel whether that somatic marker would change during the session. This made me wonder if perhaps my client's framed question (and the answer) could be found held in their body, too; and if so, then perhaps a body-scan could be a useful addition to a session in some cases. (This is another good reason for integrating Penetrating Heaven with the full Zero Balancing Protocol each time because it facilitates this body-centric way of working.)

One day a woman came to me wanting Zero Balancing purely for the relaxation. Early in the session she felt a pain in her chest. I asked if any memories or emotions were coming up, and she replied: "Yes, my partner left me last year." She started talking through what had happened as I continued to carefully place fulcrums in her lower back and ribs. Her pain quickly subsided, then she asked me: "Wait, what's the date today?" I told her, and that day happened to be the first anniversary of her partner walking out on her.

When exploring emotional pain, this "felt sense" can often be quite subtle at first, but if the client has an actual bodily pain that they can easily locate, it gives us a more obvious marker to work with.

.....

J.O., a woman with chronic pain running from her neck to her right shoulder and down into her arm, framed a question of: "Why have I got this neck/shoulder/arm issue going on?"

In her Intro Run she had the experience of "open space, empty space". The second Run then provided "a different perspective" on her current life. However, in the third Run she said: "Nothing happened!" So we had another go. This time she had the experience of "going down a tunnel with no edges", and she wiped away a tear as she got memories of her early adulthood, "bad times", which resonated with her current situation. She realised that her neck/arm pain had originated in a previous job when she was a young woman. She was currently going through similar bad times and the exact same physical pain had returned.

.....

L.B. had suffered a uterine prolapse some years ago and developed haemorrhoids. Despite different treatments and Pilates to strengthen her pelvic floor, the condition was getting worse. In her first session L.B. said she "didn't get much", except for an old memory of her father not standing up for himself. "As a young girl my dad was the source of a lot of inner angst" but she was now living back with her father and they were healing their relationship.

A month later she returned for a follow-up session. I reminded her that a memory of her dad had come up in her last session (she had forgotten this). Then I went on to explain that in Acupuncture there is a channel (The Governing Vessel) going from the pelvic floor up the backbone - the spine - to the head, and that from an Acupuncture point of view I might consider using points from this channel for her condition. She made a connection as I mentioned backbone and spine: "My dad is very gentle, and I saw him as spineless with no backbone. He wouldn't stand up for himself. When my mum died the bottom dropped out of my world." And that was when she developed the prolapse and haemorrhoids. She saw the connection.

Putting Your Finger on It

If the client has located a specific pain as the somatic marker relating to their framed issue, then it will often be responsive to touch, either by the client or, where appropriate, myself:

Pam was a young woman with a pain in her foot, but nothing showed up on her MRI scan. I discussed with her the idea that we can tend to store old emotional stress in the body, and that we could ask the question of whether there is an emotional component to her physical symptoms. This could be followed by a question to find if there is anything she needs to know (or acknowledge) about it. Her Frame Question was: “What do I need to know about the pain in my foot?”

After the Intro Run I continued with the ZB Protocol. When I was touching her foot (doing ZB fulcrums) Pam said that she suddenly got memories from her childhood, back from a time when she believed that her mum didn’t like her. And she felt very emotional about it. This opened up an opportunity for her to forgive and let go.

This illustrates that, when we frame a session with the intention of exploring the reason for physical symptoms, it can be helpful to do a Run and then spend some time touching the relevant part of the body (where appropriate), holding it with attention, because that’s where the answer may be stored.

.....

J.F. presented with a frozen shoulder, with accompanying pain and restricted movement. She had been given physiotherapy exercises which hadn’t helped much. The Bowen Technique had helped to reduce her shoulder pain, but this kept recurring because of her work as a hairdresser. We discussed how emotional stress, such as anger, grief and trauma, can be held or stored in the physical body, and that sometimes we need to acknowledge it in order to let it go. Her Frame Question was: “What do I need to know about my shoulder pain?”

I began the session with the Intro Run, then decided to gently hold her shoulder. I felt a lot of activity and movement, as if her shoulder was busy 'arguing' with itself; this seemed to be echoed by a loud chattering of sparrows outside the window. Next, I continued with the Zero Balancing Protocol and later repeated another Run of Penetrating Heaven, after which I again held her shoulder before doing some fulcrums in her upper back and neck.

J.F. said she had immediately seen her late brother. Then she had an instant realization that her frozen shoulder had started when he died suddenly of a heart attack the previous year. She also saw her mum and heard the words: "Focus on the solution, not on the problem."

This was meaningful to her and after this session her shoulder problem was resolved.

.....

Sometimes there may be a variety of different symptoms, all with a common factor: Stress.

T.A., a middle-aged man with various health problems, all of which he attributed to stress, described his session as being like a scene from the movie The Matrix "where Neo jumps up and stops in midair, and everything revolves slowly round him". (The image of the Still Point!) His interpretation: "The world is noisy and busy. But I can stop and let it revolve around me."

Seeing the connections, finding meaning and making sense of what is happening to us can be empowering, and it can help us to see our situation in a more positive light and possibly give us ideas and inspiration on what steps we may be able to take to change it.

Case Example: Integrating Two Halves

K. (Session 1)
K., a woman presenting with chronic fatigue and migraines, came for a session with me. She wanted to get to the bottom of why she had these complaints and what she could do about them.

Her Frame Question: "What is going on, or going wrong, with my body?"

As I went through each Run and the ZB Protocol, there were no obvious working signs, and nothing much appeared to be happening as K. lay with her eyes open staring at the ceiling.

Suddenly, without warning, she had an emotional release of tears and exclaimed: "Well, that's extraordinary!" (She later told me: "I thought: Well, this isn't working - and then boom!")
I said: "It's okay, just go with it. Be with it and breathe, and it will pass."
I asked if it was a memory that was coming up.
She said: "Yes, from long past."
I said: "Can you forgive the situation? Can you forgive yourself?"
She replied: "Yes, yes I think so."
"And can you see a connection?"
"Yes, but I can't quite believe it!"

Later feedback:
"It felt a bit abstract and strange as it started with colour. I experienced different colours on each side when you put pressure on my hips, dramatic red and black on the right, and soft grey and sky blue on the left. Then I had a sense of being split down the middle, or having a wall down the middle from head to toe. A self-portrait I did as an art student came up, with a mad side and a sad side. I started to see the wall dissolving and the colours mixing, and at some point I also had an image of a pure green flowing through my veins. Some Ugandan women I have recently painted came to mind (I was born there, left when I was 5). And I immediately felt it was all about Africa, where I split in two, and some battle in my body, and it made me weep. I felt great after seeing you."

K. (Session 2)

K. returned for a follow-up session and told me that leaving Uganda had been traumatic for all of her family at the time. Having received her answer of what is going on in her body, her follow-up session was to address the next steps toward health.

Her Frame Question: "What can I do about it? What is the next step?"

K. said nothing much happened in the Intro Run. And in the second Run she fell asleep. (I wondered if perhaps sleep was her answer?) In the third Run she said she had received her answer, "but it was not as dramatic as last time".

Later feedback:

"The main thing to come out of the last session was a sense that my monstrous migraine is a protective mechanism that has been erected as a barrier between me and death - like some awful parent doing its cock-eyed 'best' for their kid, causing suffering in an attempt to divert worse suffering. Does that make sense? This has meant I am owning it a bit more instead of desperately trying to separate my healthy side (me) from my sick side (not me). It feels like a move towards re-integrating the two halves. I'm doing a fair bit of visualizing this [but] I get frightened of hoping, and then getting disappointed."

Case Example: The Tree of Life

A woman in her 30s, a mother of two children, was diagnosed with abnormal cervical cells. Her periods were "all over the place" and she was bleeding a lot. She had already had a number of sessions of Penetrating Heaven with me and came to this session, one August, having just heard the news that her sister, who was pregnant, had lost her baby.

She already knew what her question was but chose not to share it with me. I opened the session with the usual Intro Run, and as I began to work on her pelvic area she started moving about on the table in obvious discomfort, crying out in pain and grief. Then she placed her hand over her lower abdomen. I hesitated but suddenly, with a sense of real urgency, I felt guided to break with the Protocol and placed my hand on top of hers, directing my attention to where she was holding. I got the impression of a baby. I imagined it was the 'memory' of a previous (full-term) pregnancy now resonating with the news of her sister's loss. I 'saw' her pelvic bowl fill up with white light, under our hands. She had a good cry, and felt relief.

After a follow-up session three months later in November, I received the following feedback:

"*Dear Gethyn,*

I felt I wanted to write to you, just to let you know the value of what you do. At times I have been most vulnerable in your treatments. You know they go deep, but they take me to the core of my being, physically, energetically, and always with angels by my side, holding my right hand. So I will tell you some of what your treatments mean to me.

As you know, it was found early in the year that I have CN2 (abnormal cervical cells), and I was offered treatment for it, which I refused. I hoped I could move forwards and heal. But it meant I was bleeding far too frequently.

At the same time, I became close to [her new partner], and our relationship grew. But sadly, and in a way that it really should not have been, I fell pregnant. It was an incredibly painful place to be, faced with such a decision. I made a choice, for my children, for [her partner], and for my own mental health. I don't really know that I would have coped with more responsibilities in my life. I've struggled in far too many ways, with divorce and single parenthood the past few years. The intense energy you felt in my abdomen was our child. I had a medical termination early in July. The physical mass passed, but I bled a little, every day, and could not move forward. I was stuck. I could not bring together my heart and my body. It was horrible. I no longer knew if I bled because of the CN2, or because I couldn't fully let go of the pregnancy.

[In the August session] I asked for help. The pain you saw in me, and what followed, was not my resonating with my sister's loss, it was my giving birth to my child - a release desperately needed for myself and this little being. It seems that neither of us could really let go, physically not pregnant, but emotionally and energetically one. We were both stagnating because my body could not hold her, and she could not leave. So I asked for help in the safe and powerfully healing space of your session. The contractions and relief of giving birth were as physically and emotionally intense as ever, I saw and felt my baby leave.

In today's session [November] I asked what comes. I cannot fully reach out to my child, she is gone to a lighter place I now know. I have to accept my choices and live with them, to find peace with this. My hand is held, and I am reassured that my child is moved on to a better place, taken care of even, by angels. She is gone now. We are unconditionally loved, always. I am able to go into my womb, it is exquisite and painful to be in that space where life is created, and denied, and everything in between. I find my uterus more freely flowing with energy, blood and vitality. It is shown to me as a tree of life, beginning to grow and blossom again.

I stopped bleeding a few weeks after the [August] session (as you would expect after giving birth), and I seem to be coming into a regular cycle now. I don't have the bleeding symptoms of CN2 anymore. It is within the unconditionally loving and healing space that your sessions allow for me that this journey of unconditional love and acceptance continues. Today I am again enveloped in pure white light, so I may become whole, unified, and a woman again. I thank you, Gethyn. From the bottom of my heart."

In that August session, I had not known the full extent of what was happening to my client. But, as I explained earlier, you don't always need to know everything. I knew enough to still be able to help her and my not knowing actually helped me to be professional and emotionally detached, which was difficult enough seeing her in such obvious pain. Thankfully, a few months later, test results showed significant improvement in her cells, and a year later she was all clear.

A Clean Slate

One day I was talking to a client, Jacqui, about how the name "Zero Balancing" came about - Fritz had had a client who said after a session that she felt "balanced back to zero" - and we discussed how sometimes in life we may feel the need to press the 'reset' button and start again. Jacqui said that in her next session she would like her Frame to explore this and to set the intention "to reset myself around a particular issue" - not to make it magically disappear but to reset her relationship with an issue in her life, to start again with it.

So we did just that. Her Frame was to reset her relationship with an old friend. The session itself was unremarkable but a few weeks later Jacqui said yes, something had changed; things were different. An old pattern of behaviour had come up in the other person, but this time Jacqui hadn't reacted in the same way. She felt that, since our session, her relationship to this person and their behaviour had changed, which was why her reaction to it had changed as well.

I felt that this "clean slate" approach could also be useful for certain health problems and started applying it in this context. One client said it was like "switching off and on again" to reset their relationship to their symptoms. Another client said: "The problem is not the pain; the problem is my relationship to the pain."

Life is all about relationship - our relationship with our self, which is then played out in our relationship to our family, friends, partner, colleagues, and the rest of the outer world.

As our relationship with our inner world improves, things in the outer world also improve.

Coming Full Circle

Penetrating Heaven began simply with “See what happens”. Then I explored the premise that the answers to our questions are within us, asking “What do I need to know?” and other variations of this question before applying it specifically to health issues in my clinic.

And although answers do come, I was surprised to find that some of my regular clients, who had successfully received answers to their questions in previous sessions, eventually stopped putting a question into their Frame, preferring instead to simply ‘dive in’ and see what happens!

So it seemed that I had come full circle. People were choosing to use the session simply to have an experience and to enjoy the journey instead of focusing on a particular destination.

Apart from practicing Penetrating Heaven in my clinic, I also offered it at summer festivals. In 2017, after a successful few days at the Into the Wild Summer Gathering, I was about to pack up my tent when a man appeared and introduced himself as Frank. We chatted about my work and he recommended a book to me: “The Unbelievable Happiness of What Is” by Jon Bernie.

Bernie explains that we have unconscious beliefs about ourselves, life, reality, and about how things ‘should’ be, but these beliefs stop us from being fully present in the moment; they get in the way and become obstacles on the path to happiness.

It makes sense that if we are coming from a place of how we believe things should be, we are not fully open to receiving the answer, and as a result our answer (or our interpretation of it) will be limited to the level of our receptivity. This is why “What do I need to know?” is such a good question because it is an invitation for more insight on the issue rather than a quest for what we think we want.

Life is fluid. We only get a snapshot of the truth that is relevant to our current situation, the next piece of the puzzle, the next step on the path, so life will always retain some of its mystery.

It is natural to seek answers to help us navigate through life. It helps us to feel in control. But as the pace of modern life has quickened we have grown used to instant gratification; access to the internet gives us information at our fingertips, and we are less comfortable with not knowing, less willing to be in the mystery and allow the story to unfold naturally. We want the answer and we want it now!

Rather than rushing to get the answer, Bernie suggests we pause and sit with the question, feel the question, feel the desire or longing behind it, the energy from which it arises. In this way you may find that the questions are more useful than the answers.

Our questions can be more than just a means to an end. They can be useful in themselves, not because they lead us to a definitive answer but because questions can open us up to more possibilities and opportunities. Questions open life up and expand our perspective whereas answers can limit or define things, bringing the energy to an abrupt full stop.

If we make 'answer getting' our focus, we can miss out on an important process of enquiry, exploration and discovery. Life is about embracing the mystery and loving what is, so instead of being attached to the result and getting the answer, if we can stay open and available and be in the present moment, we may encounter the world like a child, with innocent curiosity and imagination, free to play with ideas, and to wonder at life as it unfolds.

Zero Balancing can make you aware of neglected parts of your body. And the altered states of consciousness can make you aware of hitherto unknown parts of your psyche. In Penetrating Heaven, by putting a question into the frame, the altered states have a focus, giving the client something to relate their experience to, a context to interpret the meaning of what they encounter in their altered state.

By diving in and seeing what happens, you are diving into your self; you are meeting yourself and seeing what's there. And, like with my original journey, the experience will be personal, meaningful and relevant to your current life situation. So even if you come without a specific question, the process is still helpful and useful.

So, you can dive in and see what happens, and trust that you will receive what you need.

In Conclusion

Working with altered states of consciousness can be fascinating and transformative. I have come across many ways of doing this, among them lucid dreaming, breath-work, and shamanic practices. But working with Zero Balancing embraces the whole person: mind and body, energy and structure.

There are many paths up the mountain. This is mine, and the story of how I came across it. It has been enriching, exciting and worthwhile work.

This book focusses on one Acupuncture point, Tian Chong, GB-9, Penetrating Heaven. But I have continued to explore other points, including points on soft tissue such as the other Window of Heaven points, and Tian Fu, LU-2, Cloud Gate. I have also experimented with holding two different points together in combination, applying the same method presented in this book, and I encourage other practitioners to experiment, too. Find your own way, your own path, and follow it. The more you walk your path, the clearer and more established it becomes.

This is the end of the book but not the end of the story, and my journey continues...

Gethyn Williams

Email: penetratingheaven@gmail.com
Website: www.gethynwilliams.com

Appendix: My Method

Keys:

A light touch, which requires attention (attention amplifies the effect)
Timing: How long to hold the points for - a slow, mindful Release
Timing: How long to allow for the Run (the Pause amplifies the effect)
Get out of the way, and hold the space

FRAME: Invite the client to set an intention or a question and then suggest they let it go.

1. YOUR FIELD - Feel your feet on the floor and your body on the chair. Take a deep breath to centre yourself. Pause to set your highest intention to do your best work.

2. SPACE - Imagine a circle of privacy and protection around the table. Set the intention that the client will let go of what no longer serves them and receive what they need.

3. POSITION - Find the point, Tian Chong, GB-9. Nestle. Find the optimal level of touch.

4. PAUSE in the sweet spot - Hold, Listen, Allow. Touch with Attention.

5. ACTION - Gears: Introduce a clearer, stronger field (in you, and offer it to the client) by selecting one of the gears. Be in your fingertips at all times. Maintain the field.

6. DISCONNECT - A slow, mindful, gradual Release.

7. PAUSE for the Run - Give the client time, at least 5-10 minutes. Relax, get out of the way, trust it. Hold the space, reinforce the circle, watch for working signs, hold the field (and maintain your own field, your posture, your breath).

Gears:

(The Gears are options; you don't have to use them all)

1. Touch with Attention - Hold, Listen, Allow
2. Parallel Breaths
3. The Stillness Field
4. Silent Om
5. Heart Light
6. Bringing Down the Light from Heaven

Recommended Reading

Zero Balancing

Inner Bridges: A Guide to Energy Movement and Body Structure
Fritz Frederick Smith, MD
Humanics New Age, Atlanta, Georgia, USA,1998

The Alchemy of Touch: Moving Towards Mastery Through the Lens of Zero Balancing
Fritz Frederick Smith, MD
Complementary Medicine Press, Taos, New Mexico, USA, 2005

The Parallel Breath Meditation (DVD Video)
Fritz Smith, MD
Zero Balancing Health Association, 2012

Zero Balancing: Touching the Energy of Bone
John Hamwee
Frances Lincoln Limited, London, England, 1999

Zero Balancing Expanded: The Attitude of Awaiting a Fish
Judith Sullivan
Upledger Publications, USA, 2014

Acupuncture

A Manual of Acupuncture
Peter Deadman, Mazin Al-Khafaji, with Kevin Baker
Journal of Chinese Medicine Publications, England, 1998

Grasping the Wind: Exploration into the Meaning of Chinese Acupuncture Point Names
Andrew Ellis, Nigel Wiseman, Ken Boss
Paradigm Publications, Brookline, Massachusetts, USA, 1989

The Foundations of Chinese Medicine: A Comprehensive Text
Giovanni Maciocia
Elsevier Limited, 3rd Edition, 2015

Other

The Therapeutic Pause in Osteopathy and Manual Therapy: The Somatosensory Integration Time
Louise Tremblay
Handspring Publishing, 2015

Sabbath: Restoring the Sacred Rhythm of Rest
Wayne Muller
Bantam Doubleday Dell Publishing Group Inc, 1999

Quantum Touch: The Power to Heal
Richard Gordon
North Atlantic Books, USA, 3rd edition, 2006

Effect of Continuous Touch on Brain Functional Connectivity is Modified by the Operator's Tactile Attention
Francesco Cerritelli, Piero Chiacchiaretta, Francesco Gambi, and Antonio Ferretti of the University of Chieti-Pescara, Chieti, Italy

Stillness Speaks
Eckhart Tolle
Hodder & Stoughton, London, England, 2003

Leopard Warrior: A Journey Into The African Teachings of Ancestry, Instinct, and Dreams
John Lockley
Published by Sounds True, 2017

Love Can Open Prison Doors
Starr Daily
Arthur James Limited, England, 1947

Windows of the Mind: Exploring the Christos Technique of Mind Travel
Gerald Glaskin
Prism Press, England, 1974

The Unbelievable Happiness of What Is: Beyond Belief to Love, Fulfillment and Spiritual Awakening
Jon Bernie
Non-Duality Press, USA, 2017

Printed in Great Britain
by Amazon

72739064R00129